February 2009

Coping Successfully with Varicose Veins

Christine Craggs-Hinton, mother of three, followed a career in the Civil Service until, in 1991, she developed fibromyalgia, a chronic pain condition. Christine took up writing for therapeutic reasons and has, in the past few years, produced *Living with Fibromyalgia, The Fibromyalgia Healing Diet, The Chronic Fatigue Healing Diet, Coping with Polycystic Ovary Syndrome, Coping with Gout, How to Beat Pain, Coping with Eating Disorders and Body Image, Living with Multiple Sclerosis, Coping with Tinnitus, Coping with Hearing Loss* and, with Professor J. Hubert Lacey and Kate Robinson, *Overcoming Anorexia* (all published by Sheldon Press). She also writes for the Fibromyalgia Association UK and the related *FaMily* magazine. In recent years she has become interested in fiction writing, too.

Overcoming Common Problems Series

Selected titles

A full list of titles is available from Sheldon Press,
36 Causton Street, London SW1P 4ST and on our website at
www.sheldonpress.co.uk

Overcoming Common Problems Series

Overcoming Common Problems Series

Overcoming Common Problems

Coping Successfully with Varicose Veins

CHRISTINE CRAGGS-HINTON

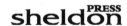

First published in Great Britain in 2008

Sheldon Press
36 Causton Street
London SW1P 4ST

The author and publisher have made every effort to ensure that the
external website and email addresses included in this book are correct and
up to date at the time of going to press. The author and publisher are not
responsible for the content, quality or continuing accessibility of the sites.

British Library Cataloguing-in-Publication Data
A catalogue record for this book is available from the British Library

ISBN 978–1–84709–015–7

1 3 5 7 9 10 8 6 4 2

Typeset by Fakenham Photosetting Ltd, Fakenham, Norfolk
Printed in Great Britain by Ashford Colour Press

Produced on paper from sustainable forests

Contents

Note: This is not a medical book and is not intended to replace advice from your doctor. Do consult your doctor if you are experiencing symptoms with which you feel you need help.

Introduction

Traditionally, varicose veins have been treated as a minor issue. It's true that varicose veins often pose more of a cosmetic concern than a real medical problem. Still, there are millions of people who are enduring symptoms that range from aching, tired legs to skin damage, ulceration and the formation of blood clots. Any condition that significantly affects the lives of a large number of people cannot, in all seriousness, be considered as 'minor'. Indeed, the complications linked with varicose veins may even be life-threatening – although only in very rare cases.

People with varicose veins can find them intensely embarrassing and go out of their way to hide their legs – particularly if they need to wear support or compression stockings. I have a chronic pain condition and often wear splints on my wrists – but society hasn't made me feel that they are ridiculous or ageing in some way. When I explain to others why I am wearing them, they show genuine concern – but that concern is often lacking when someone with varicose veins wears visible support. Varicose veins are still seen as a sign of ageing – and an ugly one at that. Unfortunately, not until the whole of the medical profession starts treating them with more seriousness will old notions finally disappear and varicose veins be treated with the consideration and respect they deserve.

If varicose veins were discovered as a new disease tomorrow and they carried no history of prejudice, the medical guidelines established would include proper investigation and treatment. It's an alarming fact, though, that as things stand, many vascular surgeons perform varicose vein operations based solely on educated guesswork rather than making use of the excellent diagnostic procedures available. As a result, all the troublesome veins are often not located and so are likely to reappear after the operation.

If you have varicose veins, this book will help you to understand what is going on in your body and inform you about the techniques of medical diagnosis currently available. You may not be aware that varicose veins can be treated – often with great success – by self-help measures such as exercise, diet, elevation of the legs and so on – all of which are discussed in this book. However, if you already have complications such as skin damage and ulceration, a surgical procedure is probably your best course of action, as explored here. Varicose veins in pregnancy and the treatment of spider veins are also tackled within these pages.

Please note that because many diseases and conditions share common symptoms it is extremely important to obtain an accurate diagnosis before following any self-help advice. If you treat yourself for the wrong illness or a specific symptom of a complex disease, you can delay legitimate treatment of a serious underlying problem. In other words, the greatest danger in self-treatment may be self-diagnosis. If you don't really know what you have, you can't treat it with any success.

1

Varicose veins – an overview

Veins that can be described as 'varicose' are twisted, lumpy and gnarled – the word 'varicose' being derived from the Latin word *varix*, meaning 'twisted'. Owing to the force of gravity, the pressure of body weight and the effort of carrying blood from the feet up to the heart, varicose veins form primarily in the legs, ankles and feet. They generally show up more easily in very pale skin and are often most visible in the calf and thigh areas, where they are close enough to the skin to be seen. While varicose veins are most common in the legs, they can also be present in the oesophagus, pelvis, uterus and rectum – haemorrhoids are a type of varicose veins.

Varicose veins – often referred to as 'varicosities' – usually develop as a result of inefficient functioning of the delicate valves in the legs, which allow the blood to 'go the wrong way' back through the vein (as described later in this chapter). Over time, the abnormal collection of blood causes the vein to become wider and lose its elasticity. It is this pooling of blood that gives varicose veins their usual dark purple or blue colouring. They can be a normal flesh colour, however.

Most varicose veins take on the appearance of bulging lengths of cord or rope and can be very unsightly, causing embarrassment and distress to the person concerned. Surprisingly, many people with varicosities experience no physical symptoms at all and their cosmetic appearance is the only downside. Others experience discomfort and pain, especially on standing and walking. In a few cases, because of the high pressure of blood in the veins at the ankle, itchy varicose eczema and darkening of the skin in that region can occur. It is the possibility of ulcers forming in the damaged skin that bothers a lot of people. The fact is, though, that ulcers only appear in a very small proportion of the varicose vein population.

It is rare for serious complications to arise with varicose veins, but they do sometimes (as explained in Chapter 3). Some people worry about a thrombosis occurring (where a dangerous blood clot called an *embolism* develops), but this seldom happens in the superficial veins that are prone to varicosities. The most dangerous thrombosis is deep vein thrombosis (also known as DVT), which arises deep beneath the surface of the skin. The only miniscule chance of a serious DVT taking place is if the varicose veins are affected by *thrombophlebitis* – a condition whereby the veins become hard and inflamed. The possible problems caused by varicose veins are discussed later in this chapter and in Chapter 3.

Modern-day treatments for varicose veins are far more sophisticated than in days gone by when the condition was not taken seriously. As a result, patients' recovery time has been reduced significantly, as has the length of a hospital stay and the cost to the National Health Service (NHS). Unfortunately, owing to the number of people affected by varicosities, there is a terrific demand for treatment. Indeed, in England and Wales, more than 50,000 surgical procedures are carried out each year on the NHS. Because varicose veins have a reputation as a minor ailment and serious medical complications are a rarity, patients with this condition are treated with lower priority than patients with certain other conditions. As a result, the waiting list for treatment can be very long.

There is no universally accepted classification for problems in the leg veins, but the one that doctors most use describes them as follows:

- varicose veins – more than 4mm wide;
- reticular varicosities (fine networks of slightly swollen veins) – less than 4mm wide;
- telangiectasia (spider veins or thread veins) – less than 1mm wide.

A number of studies have indicated that approximately 80 per cent of the population have either reticular varicosities or spider veins. (See Chapter 2 for more information on spider veins and their treatment.)

All the above-mentioned types of vein problem become more common with increasing age. The causes can include pregnancy and other hormonal changes, being overweight, an injury to the leg, sun exposure and standing for long periods, all of which are discussed in later chapters.

The early signs of varicose veins

Before the veins themselves become enlarged and twisted, an early sign of developing varicosities can include discomfort and aching in the legs after a prolonged period of standing still. There may also be cramp-like pains.

A person with early symptoms of varicose veins should seek medical advice. Self-diagnosis is not recommended because it's easy to get it wrong and so delay treatment for a more urgent problem.

Types of blood vessels

The heart is a muscular pump that transports blood around the body in tubes called arteries, capillaries and veins – all of which are referred to as 'blood vessels'. These blood vessels have the following functions.

Arteries

As the heart pumps, it pushes blood around the body through the arteries, which always take blood away from the heart. In a healthy person, arteries are larger than veins and carry oxygenated blood.

Arteries travel throughout the body, branching into smaller and smaller blood vessels. They first send the blood flow into the capillaries, then into the veins.

Capillaries

Capillaries are the smallest of the blood vessels with walls that comprise only a single layer of cells, known as the *endothelium*. The endothelium is so thin that nourishing molecules such as oxygen, water and fatty acids can pass out of the capillaries to enter the surrounding tissues. In the same way, waste products such as carbon dioxide, lactic acid and uric acid can pass through the capillary wall back into the blood to be carried away for removal from the body.

Capillaries often join together to form vessels that are a little larger, called *venules* (tiny veins).

Veins

Unlike arteries, veins always take blood towards the heart. In a healthy person, they are smaller than arteries and carry deoxygenated blood – which can be referred to as blood that has been 'used'. (It is only the pulmonary vein – the vein that takes blood away from the lungs – that carries blood that is rich in oxygen.)

Like all other blood vessels, veins are essentially hollow tubes that collapse when not filled with blood. They differ from other vessels in that they are surrounded by spiralling bands of smooth muscle that squeeze the blood and help to maintain its flow to the heart. Most veins possess fragile one-way flaps called *venous valves* that prevent gravity from causing the blood to flow backwards and pool in the lower extremities. They also have a thick outer layer of collagen – the main structure of connective tissue – which helps to maintain blood pressure and prevent blood pooling.

In the legs, movement makes the spirals of muscle around the veins squeeze the blood upwards toward the next valve. Therefore, the veins in an active person carry blood to the heart far more easily than those in an inactive person.

Because it contains less oxygen than arterial blood, the blood that flows through the veins is darker than that in the arteries. It also moves more slowly than arterial blood, and it does not pulsate.

Arterial and venous disease

There are several common diseases that affect the arteries and veins. For instance, *atherosclerosis* is characterized by the deposition of plaques of fatty material on the inner walls of the arteries. Over time, the affected arteries become choked, which can give rise to heart attacks, strokes and even gangrene of the leg. However, atherosclerosis does not cause problems in the veins, so is not linked in any way with veins becoming varicose.

Thrombosis – the clotting of blood in a blood vessel – can take place in either the arteries or veins, but is usually limited to the deep veins of the leg. As mentioned earlier, it is highly unlikely that the superficial veins near the skin – the usual site of varicosities – will develop a thrombosis.

Identifying the leg veins

In the leg, blood is carried through smaller veins that eventually join a larger one known as the *inferior vena cava*. This vein runs from the lower part of the body to the heart and lungs, carrying 'used' blood that requires oxygenating.

There are actually three types of vein in the leg, as discussed below.

Superficial veins

The first type is the *superficial vein* found just below the surface of the skin. It is often clearly visible – around the ankle, for instance – and it is usually the type of vein that is prone to become varicose.

There are two superficial veins in the leg: the *long saphenous leg vein* and the *short saphenous leg vein*. The long saphenous leg vein is the longest vein in the body, running from the foot up the inner side of the leg, to the groin. The short saphenous leg vein runs up the back of the calf to the back of the knee.

Deep veins

The second type of vein found in the leg are the *deep veins*. As the name suggests, deep veins run deep below the surface of the skin between the calf and the thigh, actually passing through the muscles of the leg. There are several deep veins and they cannot be seen.

It is in the deep veins that deep venous thrombosis can occur. However, please note that varicosities do not form in the deep veins.

Perforator veins

The third type of leg vein are the *perforator veins*, given this name because they perforate the leathery covering (called *fascia*) that surrounds the muscles of the legs. Perforators appear in a number of places in the leg and take blood from the superficial veins to the deep veins. The valves in perforators are intended only to allow blood to flow from the superficial veins into the deep veins, but if the valves become weak and stop working, blood is pushed back into the superficial veins. The result can be high blood pressure in the superficial veins, as well as the onset of varicosities.

All the veins in the legs contain delicate valves that enable:

- blood to flow upwards towards the heart; or
- blood to flow from the superficial veins to the deep ones, via the perforating veins.

The normal action of blood vessels in the legs

The heart is responsible for sending blood to every single cell in the body. It is also responsible for pumping blood to the lungs, where the carbon dioxide build-up is removed from the blood, and oxygen taken on board.

In the legs, oxygenated blood is moved by gravity down the legs and into the feet. The blood must then return to the heart to become oxygenated again, a function that is achieved by a pumping movement performed by the muscles in the legs – the muscles actually squash the veins and force the blood upwards and into the torso (as described in more detail below). When the muscles relax and the veins open again, the blood would rush back down the leg – a problem called reflux – if valves that act like one-way flaps were not present to prevent this from occurring.

Leg valves that work efficiently protect the legs and can be described as 'competent'.

Valves in the leg veins

Obviously, blood returns to the heart far more easily when we are lying down. It needs to work against gravity, however, when we are standing upright, for the heart is then positioned a good distance above the feet.

Because of gravity and the weight of blood in the arteries, the act of standing increases the pressure of the blood flow from the heart to the feet. This is called *gravitational* or *hydrostatic* pressure and aids the blood flow down from the heart to the legs. This same gravitational or hydrostatic pressure ensures, however, that there is not sufficient pressure in the blood in the veins for it to return to the heart. In fact, standing still for a long time can cause the blood to stagnate so much that it fails to reach the brain and the person may even faint.

The fact that we don't usually faint when we stand for a long time means that blood does usually return to the heart, from where it is then sent up to the brain. This is because, in the legs, the muscles push the blood upwards from the ankle and lower leg into the torso, as mentioned earlier. This pump system is sometimes known as the 'muscle pump' or 'peripheral heart'.

When the muscle pump is working efficiently, the movement of the muscles in the leg pushes on the veins and squashes them so that the blood in the vein moves upwards. Without the valves, the

Blood flowing
to heart

Healthy valve
prevents reverse
blood flow

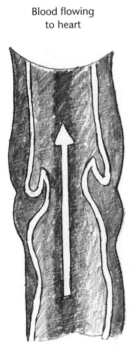
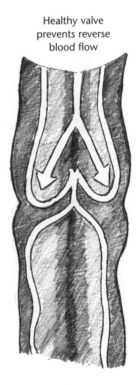

Figure 1   Normal one-way vein valves

blood would move without any particular direction – it certainly wouldn't be pushed up toward the torso. Furthermore, the pressure of blood in the ankles and feet would be immense.

In the main superficial veins of the legs, a valve is positioned at every 5–10cm (see Fig. 1).

When the valves fail

Weak and damaged valves in any of the leg veins mean that the muscle pump cannot do its job properly, and so it squeezes a smaller amount of blood upwards than it should – a situation that is particularly harmful if the veins at the knee are affected. Over time, the vein walls weaken and the pressure of blood in the veins causes some of the blood to flow downwards, away from the heart. Gradually, the weakened veins lose their elasticity and become

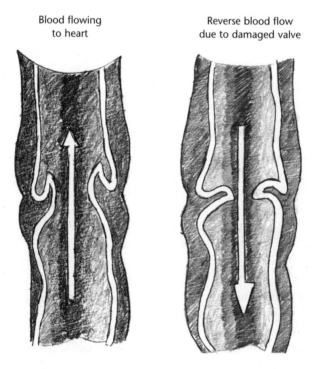

Blood flowing to heart

Reverse blood flow due to damaged valve

Figure 2   Varicose vein valves

longer and wider. This, of course, leads to space constraints, because these bulkier veins still need to occupy the same space as if they were a normal size. To fit this space, the veins twist and fold, often appearing as snake-like bulges beneath the skin. These enlarged and twisted veins have now become *varicose*.

If not dealt with early, varicose veins do slowly worsen over time. The widening of the affected vein pulls the valve cusps further and further apart so that valve after valve becomes incompetent down the leg, as shown in Figure 2. The continuous downward flow of blood makes the vein enlarge further, its appearance becoming more bulky and pronounced beneath the skin.

There is an array of symptoms associated with varicose veins. They are discussed later in this chapter.

Which veins can become varicose?

When the valves are inefficient in the perforator veins, blood is pushed out under high pressure into the superficial veins, which often leads to varicosities. Note that it only takes one faulty valve to produce a varicose vein.

The saphenous veins most commonly become varicose.

The long saphenous vein

Given the right circumstances, it is the *long saphenous vein* and its tributaries that most often become varicose. In most people, this vein is evident when they stand up, it being the one on the inner side of the ankle, just in front of the bone. It travels up the inner side of the calf and thigh to the groin, where it becomes submerged in order to join the main deep vein, the *femoral vein*.

The short saphenous vein

The *short saphenous vein*, the other main vein beneath the skin of the leg, together with its tributaries, can also become varicose – but not so commonly as the long saphenous vein. The short saphenous vein starts behind the bone on the outer side of the ankle and travels up the back of the calf before submerging to join the main deep vein just above and behind the knee. The exact location of the vein in the knee area varies from person to person. Indeed, its site should be checked by ultrasound scan before any surgical procedure is carried out on it.

Other veins

Varicose veins can develop in other veins in the leg, without valve problems in the long saphenous vein, the short saphenous vein or the perforator veins. Fortunately, these varicose veins are usually quite small and cause few symptoms, if any at all.

Varicose veins versus spider veins

Some people confuse varicose veins with spider veins (sometimes called 'thread veins'), believing the latter are as troublesome as the former. Spider veins are indeed a smaller version of varicose veins, but they occur in the capillaries only – the smallest blood vessels in the body. Spider veins are usually red or blue in colour, they resemble tiny tree branches or spider webs with their short, jagged lines and they are commonly found on the face and legs, closer to the surface of the skin than varicose veins. They can cover either a very small or very large area of skin, but they rarely produce symptoms. However, spider veins can pose a cosmetic problem, particularly when they develop on the face.

As with varicose veins, a back-up of blood can produce spider veins. They can also be inherited or caused by hormonal changes (see 'What causes valve failure', page 15). Spider veins can also result from exposure to the sun, especially in a fair-skinned person. In this instance, they are likely to appear across the cheeks and on the nose.

Varicose veins – the signs and symptoms

As well as visible, enlarged veins, the most common signs and symptoms of varicose veins in the legs and feet include the following, as found in the important Edinburgh Vein Study:[1]

- a feeling of heaviness;
- legs that tire easily;

- an aching pain;
- cramps;
- swelling;
- numbness;
- restless leg syndrome;
- itching and tingling, often related to an irritated rash – see *Venous eczema*, page 27;
- darkening of the skin;
- skin ulcers, often near the ankle.

People who have varicose veins often complain of aching and heaviness and a feeling of tension in their legs, particularly after standing still for a long time. They may also experience itching and the sensation of heat and tenderness over the trouble spots, which worsens as the day wears on.

Interestingly, in a study of over 1,500 people with varicose veins, it was concluded that in men the majority of lower limb symptoms probably have a non-venous cause. In other words, it seems that varicose veins are not, by any means, always responsible for lower limb aches and pains.[2] We know that varicose veins don't always cause symptoms, and therefore it can be assumed that only the most severe cases give rise to aching and similar problems. In addition, the study found that, in women, the only symptoms that correlated strongly with the presence of varicose veins were heaviness, tension, aching and itching. The existence of varicose veins was not significantly linked with restless legs, cramping, swelling or tingling. It makes sense, then, to say that before attributing any leg symptoms you may have to varicose veins, your doctor should attempt to ascertain whether there may be another problem.

It is usually possible to tell whether varicose veins are the cause of symptoms by wearing good support stockings. If the aching and other symptoms disappear, it's fairly safe to say that varicose veins were the cause. Don't rely on this test, though. Any symptoms in any part of the body should be 'officially' diagnosed by your doctor.

Further research is needed into the symptoms associated with varicose veins. The size of the varicosities is not always an indication of their potential for causing symptoms.

If you are not sure whether the aching, heaviness and other symptoms in your legs are severe enough to warrant treatment, ask your doctor to refer you to a vascular surgeon. When the surgeon has explained the procedures that may offer most benefit in your case, it is up to you to weigh up whether your veins are indeed troublesome enough for you to put yourself through a surgical procedure with its inconvenience and risks. If you have another condition that affects your legs – arthritis, for example – you should accept that this may be the main source of your leg problems. Wearing good support stockings for a couple of weeks will help you to determine whether the chief culprit is your varicose veins or your other health condition.

See Chapter 3 for a discussion of other symptoms of varicose veins.

Who gets varicose veins?

Estimates of the incidence of varicose veins vary enormously. Some experts are of the opinion that, in Western-style, industrialized societies, the condition affects approximately 19 per cent of men and 36 per cent of women, but others believe the figures are more like 45 per cent of men and 55 per cent of women. Whatever the reality of the matter, varicose veins are undeniably very common. People usually get varicose veins between the ages of 30 and 70. They can, however, develop in younger people, particularly in women during pregnancy.

Other factors that can increase a person's chances of developing the condition include:

- Hormonal factors: as noted above, more women than men have varicose veins. This is thought to be due to hormonal factors, as described below. Some experts believe that as much as three-quarters of the female population have or will develop varicose veins, whereas only one-quarter of men have or will develop them. I reiterate that there are no conclusive figures of incidence, however.
- Dietary and other lifestyle factors: studies carried out on the prevalence of varicose veins show that they are less common

in the developing world than in industrialized societies. For example, only 2 per cent of the female population in rural India have varicose veins, and only 5 per cent have them in central and eastern Africa. This may largely be due to dietary factors – people in the developing world tend to eat foods in their natural state whereas in the developed world we eat too many processed foods. A diet lacking in fibre can also put a person at higher risk of varicose veins, and consuming a lot of salt can cause swelling and water retention and make varicosities worse. Exercise is also likely to be a factor – in the developed world we tend to use our cars more than our feet. (See Chapter 6 for more information on diet, and Chapter 5 for more information on exercise.)

- Ageing: although varicose veins can occur in teenagers, the condition is more likely to develop with increasing age. This is because ageing creates wear and tear of the valves in the veins, raising the likelihood of malfunction over time.
- Genetic factors: having family members with varicose veins seems to make an individual more prone to developing them (see 'Genetics' below).
- Prolonged standing: varicose veins are more likely to occur in people who stand up at work, particularly for long periods.
- Tight clothing: wearing tight clothing, such as corsets, tights or belts, can lead to the onset of varicose veins.

What causes valve failure?

Varicose veins develop as a result of incompetence in one or more of the valves in the leg, leading to a knock-on effect in other leg valves. We don't fully understand why the incompetence occurs in the first place, but there are a few theories on the matter, as discussed below.

Genetics

Our veins are largely composed of a substance called *collagen*, which gives them their strength, and a substance called *elastin*, which gives them their elasticity. A number of studies have indicated, however, that these substances are abnormal in people with varicose veins.

As a result, the muscle pump fails to push sufficient blood upwards toward the torso.

Interestingly, research into vein weakness and varicose veins in siblings has indicated a link to a particular faulty gene.[3] Varicose veins certainly appear to 'run in the family', which strengthens the theory of a genetic component.

The theory of a genetic factor would seem to apply, most of all, to the usual type of varicose vein that develops for no obvious reason.

Hormonal factors

As stated earlier, women are more likely to have varicose veins than men. This is believed to be due largely to the hormonal changes a woman experiences during her lifetime. In fact, studies have shown that a woman who has had children is more likely to develop varicose veins, and that the risk of them arising is raised from the first trimester (period of 3 months) of the pregnancy. It appears that women are also more at risk during the menopause, in the last 14 days of their menstrual cycle each month, and if they take oestrogen or progesterone in the contraceptive pill or oestrogen as hormone replacement therapy (HRT). In all these cases, women have higher than normal levels of the female hormones circulating in their blood, and this has the effect of relaxing the smooth muscle of the vein walls and therefore impeding the muscle pump.

Pregnancy is a particularly hazardous time for the veins, for not only are there high levels of circulating progesterone in the bloodstream, but there is also a huge increase in the amount of blood in the body, which can cause the veins to stretch. The growing baby increases the pressure on the leg veins, too. Fortunately, after a woman's first pregnancy, varicose veins usually improve 3–12 months after the birth of the child. Improvement may not be seen after subsequent pregnancies, and an increased number of abnormal veins can appear each time.

In a small percentage of women, a condition known as 'milk leg' can arise during pregnancy. This comes about when the circulating hormones actually destroy the leg valves and the pressure of the pooled blood in the leg causes significant swelling.

There is a more in-depth discussion on pregnancy and the veins in Chapter 4.

Prolonged standing or sitting

Standing or sitting for long periods can also be a cause of valve failure and varicosities. Such prolonged maintenance of one position raises the pressure on the leg veins and exerts great stress on the valves. Sitting with your legs crossed or bent up beneath you means the veins have to work extra hard to pump up the blood to your heart. Some people are so affected by the aching and pain from their varicose veins that their ability to walk or stand for any length of time is seriously impaired. Fortunately, this only happens in severe cases.

Soldiers on long marches and standing on guard duty are taught how to help the muscle pump to work. They do this by repeatedly tightening and relaxing their calf muscles to aid the upward movement of blood. If they fail to do this, the pooling of blood in their legs can cause them to faint, particularly on a hot day when the veins are already dilated.

For support and protection, soldiers used to wear puttees, which were long strips of cloth wound spirally around their legs from the calf to the ankle. This is believed to have helped the muscle pump to push up blood through the veins during long marches.

Being overweight

Because being overweight exerts added pressure on the venous system, overweight people are believed to be at higher risk of developing varicose veins. It would appear that the heavier a person is, the more pressure there is on the veins and the more likely they are to become varicose.

As yet, studies on obesity and varicose veins have shown inconsistent results and there is a need for further investigation.

Diet and bowel habit

Experts have suggested that lack of fibre in the diet and constipation – which leads to sitting and straining on the toilet – is one of the leading causes of varicose veins. Constipation can restrict the flow of blood as it returns upwards to the body through the deep veins in the legs, and straining to move the bowel closes off the veins. The blood backs up and is forced to take another course, passing instead through the superficial veins, where an excess of blood eventually causes the veins to become varicose.

See Chapter 6 for details of how to increase your fibre intake and information on other dietary recommendations for varicose veins.

Damage to the leg

A prior surgical procedure or trauma of some kind to the leg – an accident, for example – can interrupt the normal blood flow process and lead to varicose veins.

Cosmetic embarrassment

We live in a society in which women feel pressured to be slim and attractive with nice-looking legs. Many women with varicose veins feel they must hide their legs by always wearing trousers, thick tights or long skirts – but in so doing they are giving in to the pressures and allowing how they feel about their physical appearance to dictate what they wear and even the activities they indulge in. Dislike of one's outer self can quite easily give rise to depression and all that that entails. I understand, however, that it is simpler to cover the problem than find the strength to overcome the extreme upset and embarrassment it causes. Guess what, though? Many of the people you are hiding your legs from have varicose veins themselves.

It is known that our body image is crucial to our happiness and our state of health. Therefore taking steps to create a positive body image is highly recommended. Using biofeedback, relaxation and the stress-busting suggestions (see Chapter 10) can make a difference to how you feel about your appearance. If these things don't help, give hypnotherapy a serious try (as discussed on page 106). Don't forget, too, that there are several non-surgical means of improving the appearance of varicose veins – even of encouraging them to disappear in some cases. These include following a healthy, nutritious diet, taking regular exercise, using the recommended herbal remedies and trying certain complementary therapies – all of which are explored in this book.

In general, men are not so badly affected as women by cosmetic pressures, but, even so, many avoid wearing shorts on holiday and on the tennis court or sports field. Obviously, men too can improve the appearance of their veins by following the self-help treatment in this book.

Surgery may be offered to a person who is very troubled by the look of his or her veins – but this is not always the case. Some people exaggerate their varicose vein symptoms in order to be offered a removal procedure.

Haemorrhoids

Haemorrhoids (commonly known as 'piles') are swollen blood vessels – much like varicose veins, but they are located in the rectal area. More than half of the UK population experience haemorrhoids at some point in their lives. They are common in all ages, particularly in pregnant women.

Haemorrhoids are believed to be linked to excess pressure in the anus and lower rectum, caused by such things as straining on the toilet to pass a hard stool, poor blood circulation, heavy lifting or being overweight.

The symptoms of irritation and swelling can be relieved by the following:

- taking regular warm baths;
- consuming a high-fibre diet (i.e. with plenty of wholegrain cereals, fruit and vegetables) – much as described in Chapter 6;
- drinking plenty of fluids, especially water, to keep bowel movements soft;
- using ice packs in the affected area (avoid applying them directly to the skin);
- taking a gentle laxative – but only when absolutely necessary;
- applying soothing over-the-counter creams or local anaesthetic to the area;
- using prescription products that aim to reduce pain and inflammation.

To remove haemorrhoids, there are several non-surgical procedures available, as well as, in severe cases, surgical removal.

If you think you have haemorrhoids, you should visit your doctor.

2

Spider veins

In the Caucasian (white) population, at least half of all adult females – particularly fair-skinned ones – are bothered by the cosmetic appearance of spider veins (also known as thread veins, star-bursts, flare veins and matted veins). They are visible as small clusters of tiny veins that are red, blue or purple in colour, and they may be present on the face, neck, upper arms, ankles, calves and thighs. Although these super-fine spider veins lie close to the surface of the skin and are connected with the larger venous system, they are by no means an essential part of it.

Spider veins are also known as *'spider angioma'* or *'spider telangiectasia'*. They are harmless to your health, may come and go, and are usually symptom-free. In a few cases, however, the person experiences a feeling of heat or throbbing in lower limb spider veins, as well as cramping pains and swelling. Very rarely, spider veins are related to a more serious problem such as skin damage. Contrary to popular belief, facial telangiectasia are not linked to excessive alcohol intake.

Spider veins can arise because of:

- the presence of a condition called 'rosacea', in which the facial blood vessels become enlarged;
- certain medications such as cortisone creams;
- heredity – they may run in the family;
- elevated oestrogen levels that occur during pregnancy;
- taking hormone replacement therapy (HRT) during menopause;
- exposure to oestrogen-mimicking substances such as certain pesticides and petrochemicals;
- a condition called 'oestrogen dominance' in which there are elevated levels of oestrogen;
- fibrocystic breast disease.

If you are taking an oestrogen-based therapy and have developed spider veins, ask your doctor if you can reduce the dose.

In some people, particularly women, spider veins can become evident in the teenage years. For others they may be more of a cosmetic problem as they reach their 40s. Younger people tend to be very conscious of their appearance and hate any physical imperfection that picks them out from the rest of the crowd. Even quite a small starburst on the back of the calf can cause significant distress, made even worse when friends point it out. Often the imperfection is greater in the person's mind than it really is and can even lead to depression.

As noted above, women are more likely to have spider veins than men, owing chiefly to hormonal factors. Moreover, in men, spider veins on the lower limbs are not nearly as evident because they are usually covered by hair growth. In today's world, women feel the need to be as slim and attractive as possible, causing them to tend to be far more troubled than men by the appearance of spider veins. For that reason, they may be offered treatment more readily. However, if a man hates the appearance of his spider veins, treatment may be an option. Unfortunately, whether or not a person is offered treatment can also depend on the area he or she lives in. Spider veins usually fall into one of three basic patterns:

- a true spider shape with groups of veins radiating outwards from a dark central point – this pattern can be present in any of the common sites for such veins;
- resembling the branches of a tree – this pattern is commonly seen on the outer thigh;
- thin separate lines – such 'linear' lines are usually seen on the inner knee.

Symptoms associated with spider veins

Spider veins are quite different from varicose veins. As mentioned in Chapter 1, varicose veins are larger and darker in colour and have a bulging, twisted appearance. Being smaller, spider veins are far less likely to cause discomfort and seldom lead to complications. The main symptoms related to spider veins on the lower limbs include aching, burning, swelling and night cramps. However, symptoms are so rare that further investigation is likely to be carried out to ensure that varicose veins are not also present. (See Chapter 7 for information on testing for varicose veins.)

Facial spider veins are normally tiny enough to preclude symptoms.

Microsclerotherapy

As discussed in Chapter 8, sclerotherapy is often the treatment of choice for varicose veins. It is also frequently used for improving the appearance of spider veins, with very fine needles being used. A typical microsclerotherapy session involves the patient lying down on an examination couch and the skin over the spider veins being cleaned with antiseptic. The doctor then injects a special chemical solution into the affected veins – on average, one injection is administered for every inch of spider vein, which can mean up to 40 injections in one session. You can expect to feel a slight burning sensation as each needle is inserted. The liquid chemical causes the vein walls to swell, stick together and seal up, eventually to be absorbed by the body.

After the procedure, a cotton wool ball is secured into place by a strip of compression tape over every injection site, and you are likely to be asked to wear compression stockings for at least 3 days. In the first few days after microsclerotherapy, some people experience leg cramps – a temporary situation that requires no treatment. Some treated veins may actually look worse before they begin to look better. When the compression stockings are removed, there may also be some reddening and slight bruising at the injection sites, but this should disappear within a month. In some cases, areas of brown pigmentation may remain for up to a year before fading.

Because there is a very slight risk of clots forming in the deep veins of the legs after microsclerotherapy treatment, you are likely to be advised to take a 20-minute brisk walk shortly after the procedure. Thereafter, in the long term, you should try to keep generally active, avoiding prolonged sitting, standing, squatting, heavy lifting and any 'pounding' type of exercise, including jogging.

Many people require repeated microsclerotherapy treatments, at intervals of approximately 1 month. The appearance of your legs will be more noticeably improved after each session. In general, microsclerotherapy makes the skin appear younger, clearer and more healthy-looking, and most people are pleased with the result.

Unfortunately, injection microsclerotherapy cannot prevent new spider veins from arising in the future. You may find that in time you need 'touch-ups' or full treatments for new veins. If you prefer not to have further treatments, your legs will still look better than if you had never had the treatment.

Laser therapy

Laser therapy is generally used on veins that are too tiny for microsclerotherapy treatment. It is very effective for removing spider veins on the face, but not always successful for those on the legs.

The use of a laser to remove spider veins is easy, fast and effective, and it has been popular for over 30 years. Research has developed many types of laser, all of which use a focused beam of light to heat up the vein, collapse the vein walls and cause the vein to disappear – the same principle as used in sclerotherapy and microsclerotherapy. Before the laser or light source is used, the skin over the affected area is cooled by chilled air or the application of a gel. This reduces discomfort and lowers the risk of skin reddening.

During laser therapy, a small laser hand piece called a 'fibreoptic laser cable' delivers a precise dosage of energy to a targeted vein in a series of short pulses that heats the vein up. The blood and walls of the blood vessels absorb the energy, making the blood clot and eventually be absorbed by the body. The laser 'traces' individual vessels, and the pulses feel like tiny 'snaps', similar to the flick of a small elastic band. The sensations are well tolerated by most patients – however, if it is found to be painful, an anaesthetic cream may be used to numb the area. The procedure is usually carried out on an out-patient basis and takes only 10–20 minutes.

Laser therapy should cause the treated veins to disappear within two to three treatment sessions, which are likely to be spaced at intervals of 3–6 weeks. If new spider veins emerge some time after treatment, additional treatments will give a better result. It is unrealistic, though, to expect that every single spider vein will disappear. Patients can look forward to a general improvement of appearance and therefore raised self-esteem.

Laser therapy can cause the skin to redden temporarily – this redness disappears within a couple of days. In some cases, bruising occurs, but this disappears within a few weeks. Most patients are pleased with the results in a very short time, but the final outcome may not be apparent for several months.

When the blood vessels are too small or too numerous to trace, an ultrasound scanner can be used to treat the whole area. There is also now a 'large spot' 10mm laser that facilitates the treatment of large areas.

Cryotherapy

Meaning literally 'cold therapy', cryotherapy is a traditional procedure used to destroy tissue by repeatedly freezing and thawing it. The most commonly used freezing source is liquid nitrogen. However, this treatment is not always satisfactory in that scarring can occur.

Cauterization

In cauterization, burning is used to remove or close a part of the body. In the case of spider veins, a small instrument employs heat to seal the tiny blood vessels during surgery. It is important that you stay out of the sun until the area has completely healed. Cauterization can leave scarring, however, so it is becoming a less popular treatment.

3

Possible complications
of varicose veins

Although most varicose veins are not dangerous and are actually symptom-free, the more severe ones can lead to complications if they are not treated. These complications are due to excessive blood pooling and poor blood circulation throughout the affected limb.

People with problems in their deep veins are more likely to experience complications. However, deep vein problems are rare.

Ankle swelling

In a few people, varicose veins can cause the ankles to swell. This is because on standing, walking or sitting with your feet on the ground, the pressure of excess blood and other fluids in the veins results in fluid being squeezed out of the tissues. Fortunately, in most cases, swelling related to varicose veins disappears after a night in bed. However, the presence of varicose veins is not the only reason for the ankles to swell, and your doctor will need to carry out a thorough investigation to determine the cause. Some people find that their ankles are still swollen after their veins have been surgically treated. If the swelling remains for more than 3 months after surgery, it's safe to say that varicose veins are not the cause.

Lipodermatosclerosis (skin damage)

Strangely, many people with large varicose veins manage to avoid skin damage whereas a few people with smaller varicose veins encounter a lot of skin damage – and as yet it is not known why. It is estimated that, overall, only 6 per cent of people with varicosities are troubled with skin problems.

Damage to the skin can be caused by very high pressure of blood in the leg veins, which in turn can lead to the development of ulcers. As a rule, the discoloration first appears in the form of brownish pigmentation in blotchy patches, and it later change to a dark, shiny brown. The correct medical term for this phenomenon is *lipodermatosclerosis* – *lipo* meaning fat, *dermato* meaning relating to the skin, and *sclerosis* meaning hardening and scarring.

If you are wondering where 'fat' comes into the equation, it's because it is not just the skin that becomes discoloured and damaged, but also the fatty layer beneath that turns hard and shrinks. Eventually, the area affected takes on a dented appearance and the whole leg just above the ankle can become thinner and pitted – a further cause of cosmetic concern.

Treatment

People with lipodermatosclerosis, or skin damage (also referred to as 'skin changes') need to seek medical attention to prevent the condition from worsening. If you would rather not undergo surgery or a less invasive procedure called sclerotherapy (in which a solution is injected into the vein to cause the vein walls to stick together, as discussed in Chapter 8), you may be able to improve the condition of the skin by wearing graduated compression stockings (see Chapter 5). If the skin problems worsen despite use of such stockings, it may be advisable for sclerotherapy or vein stripping to be carried out (see Chapters 8 and 9). Discuss your options with your vascular surgeon.

Venous eczema

Venous eczema – also known as *varicose eczema, gravitational eczema* or *stasis dermatitis* – commonly arises in varicose lower limbs, usually just above the ankle, on the inside of the leg. It is caused by insufficient blood being pushed back up the leg and subsequent pooling of the blood (known as 'stasis'). Poor return of blood to the groin area increases pressure in the capillaries, with the result that fluid and red blood cells can 'leak' out into the skin. The red blood cells eventually break down, causing the skin to become brown in colour and maybe to crack. It also weakens the skin in this area, making it thin and papery and prone to bruising and ulceration.

Treatment

If left untreated, venous eczema can become severe, causing redness and inflamed, scaly skin to stretch around a large area of the lower leg. An emollient may help. Treatment of venous eczema usually includes topical applications of corticosteroid-based creams. However, such creams are not recommended for long-term use because they can make the skin thinner and more fragile. Compression stockings are another alternative – they help to push the underlying build-up of fluids back out of the lower leg. Unfortunately, compression stockings do not always stop the problem, and your vascular surgeon may recommend a surgical procedure to seal up or remove the veins (see Chapters 8 and 9).

Atrophie blanche

Where skin damage is severe, shiny white patches appear over the areas of darker pigmentation. This is known by the French phrase *atrophie blanche*.

Cellulitis

Unfortunately, the cracks and general poor state of the skin makes it liable to developing a bacterial infection. A condition known as *cellulitis* can then spread through the leg. Cellulitis is a potentially serious bacterial infection that can attack superficial tissues as well as tissues underlying the skin. If left untreated, cellulitis can cause a venous ulcer to form. It can even spread into the bloodstream, travel to the lymph nodes and become a life-threatening condition.

If you recognize any of the following signs and symptoms of cellulitis, you should seek urgent medical attention:

- reddened skin;
- swelling;
- tenderness;
- a feeling of heat in the affected area.

In addition, over time, the area of redness is likely to expand and small red spots may form on top of the affected area. Occasionally, small blisters may develop and burst.

Treatment

The mainstay of treatment for cellulitis is antibiotic medication. Your doctor will prescribe the type he or she thinks will be most effective. If the first course of medication fails to work, don't hesitate to return to your doctor.

Superficial thrombophlebitis

Sometimes referred to simply as *phlebitis*, *thrombophlebitis* is present when a vein becomes inflamed and a blood clot (a *thrombosis*) forms inside the inflamed section. The condition affects the superficial veins, particularly those that are varicose, making the skin over them feel sensitive, swollen and inflamed. The person may also develop a high temperature. The veins and skin usually return to normal after a period of 2–6 weeks.

Superficial thrombophlebitis can arise after a slight injury to the vein, such as occurs after having intravenous injections or infusions in hospital, or in people who self-inject 'street drugs'. Scratching an itchy area or grazing it can also create a slight injury that leads to superficial thrombophlebitis. In addition, veins can be damaged by certain rare disorders, such as Mondor's disease, Buerger's disease and Behçet's disease.

An abnormality in a blood clotting factor can make it more likely for a blood clot to occur in a vein that is inflamed. The conditions that can alter clotting factors in the blood include:

- pregnancy (see page 37);
- childbirth – it has been estimated that one in 200 women experience an episode of thrombophlebitis in the leg within 48 hours of giving birth;
- smoking;
- the contraceptive pill;
- an hereditary blood disorder that causes blood clots to develop more easily than they should;
- cancer.

If you suffer from recurring bouts of superficial thrombophlebitis, you should ask your doctor for tests to be carried out. The condition can be an early indication of a more serious disorder, such as some of those mentioned above. Fortunately, it is very rare for cancer to first show itself as thrombophlebitis.

Treatment

If the symptoms are relatively mild, the condition may resolve itself without treatment in the space of a few weeks. Whether symptoms are mild or severe, you can help to ease the pain and swelling in the following ways:

- place a hot flannel (as hot as you can comfortably bear) over the troublesome area;
- raise the affected leg so that your foot is higher than your hip when you are sitting. You can also lie on the sofa with your leg raised on cushions. In bed, keep your leg raised by resting it on a couple of pillows;
- take anti-inflammatory painkillers such as ibuprofen, aspirin or paracetamol, as prescribed by your doctor. If you are pregnant, ask your doctor for advice regarding medications;
- alternatively, apply topical ointments such as hirudoid cream, which contains a compound called heparinoid. Hirudoid cream helps to dissolve any blood clots, reduce inflammation and improve the blood supply to the skin. It is available on prescription from your doctor;
- wear good compression (support) stockings (see Chapter 5 for more information on support stockings). Your doctor may be able to prescribe these.

When the inflammation has settled, it is recommended that you see your doctor for advice regarding treatment to seal up or remove your varicose veins. In some cases, good comes from bad when the affected varicose veins remain blocked and slowly shrivel up. This removes the need for surgical intervention.

Deep vein thrombosis

Research has shown that a very small number of people with superficial thrombophlebitis go on to develop a thrombosis in the deep veins – a deep vein thrombosis or DVT. However, such DVTs are seldom serious in nature. A blood clot (from thrombophlebitis) can also occur in the long saphenous vein, in the area near the groin where the long saphenous vein and the deep veins meet. To prevent the risk of a severe DVT at the groin, the vein is likely to require tying off as a matter of urgency.

When superficial thrombophlebitis develops in a vein that was previously normal, not varicose, DVT is a possibility. If you experience any of the following, you should visit your doctor immediately:

- redness, hardness and inflammation spreading up the inner thigh towards the groin;
- sudden considerable swelling of the whole leg;
- the onset of breathing problems (or worsening of them if you already suffer from this problem);
- chest pains.

The last two of these symptoms are listed because it is possible for a blood clot to travel up from the leg to the lungs.

The chances of a DVT occurring are very slim. Indeed, it is estimated that only between one and three people per 1,000 in the UK develop the condition each year. If it does happen, treatment aims to prevent the following:

- the blood clot growing larger;
- a piece of the clot breaking off and travelling to the lungs;
- the development of further clots;
- post-thrombotic syndrome, which occurs when an obstruction remains in the vein, giving rise to pain, an accumulation of fluid (oedema), greater intensity of skin pigmentation and leg ulceration.

The most common drug treatment is anticoagulant medication, which stops blood clots forming so easily and prevents new ones from developing. Warfarin or heparin are typically used. Note that there is some concern that drinking cranberry juice can interfere with the way warfarin works.

Other complications

Other complications can arise as a result of superficial thrombophlebitis:

- Infection – a bacterial infection can sometimes arise in the affected vein, resulting in more redness, increased pain and a feeling of being unwell. The best treatment for a bacterial infection in the veins is a course of prescription antibiotics from your doctor. In rare instances, the infection becomes severe and spreads to other parts of the body; however, the use of antibiotics will usually prevent this.
- Damaged skin – occasionally, a permanent blood clot will completely block the inside of the vein, giving rise to post-thrombotic syndrome, as mentioned above. Superficial thrombophlebitis can also cause the skin to become hard and scarred.
- After surgery – varicose veins can be linked with a higher risk of developing DVT after pelvic or abdominal surgery. However, during the surgery, surgeons take extra care to reduce the risk of DVT, as a result of which there is very rarely a problem.

Venous ulcers

Also known as abcesses, boils, pustules and carbuncles, ulcers can be very painful and are among the more severe complications of varicose veins. A venous ulcer is an open sore of the skin. Venous ulcers are usually caused by a minor wound such as an abrasion that occurs on scratching an itch in an area of skin damage. The open sore is generally maintained by inflammation and poor blood flow to the area. Slow healing due to lipodermatosclerosis (see pages 26–7) is also a factor.

Research has indicated that only 0.2 per cent of the population develop venous ulcers as a result of varicose veins, 40–50 per cent of which are due to poor blood flow and incompetent perforating veins.

Venous ulcers have a raw base, which may look pink and clean. However, the open wound may attract a bacterial infection, making the base appear yellow and filling it with pus. Common locations for leg ulcers are around the shin or ankle. If they develop higher in the leg, they are likely to have a cause other than varicose veins. Venous ulcers may be either large or small and either pain-free or very painful. The painful ones tend to become increasingly more troublesome towards the end of the day.

Infected ulcers

Venous ulcers are slow to heal and commonly develop a bacterial infection, which should be treated with a 2-week course of broad-spectrum penicillin or other antibiotics. The additional use of topical antibiotics (in the form of creams, for example) should be avoided, owing to the risk of increasing bacterial resistance.

Initial treatment

The application of a compression bandage around the affected area can reduce pressure in the superficial veins and so encourage an ulcer to heal. Your doctor or nurse may use a single and multilayer elastic bandage system, a short stretch bandage or an elasticated tubular bandage (Tubigrip, for example). Compression by means of a pneumatic device (Flowtron, for example) can also promote healing – ask your doctor about this. However, if side-effects such as tingling, numbness, pain or darkened toes occur, you should remove the compression straight away and see your doctor once more.

Further management

When a venous ulcer has healed, it is recommended that you follow some simple advice aimed at preventing its recurrence. It has been reported that the recurrence rate of venous leg ulcers can be greatly reduced by adhering to the following guidelines:

- using good compression (support) stockings;
- taking care of your skin, by using moisturizing creams and so on;
- frequently elevating your legs when sitting and raising the foot of your bed so that your legs are higher than your trunk when in bed;
- performing calf exercises, such as going up and down on your toes several times a day and perhaps carrying out a 'step' exercise on the bottom step of your stairs, or with a step-aerobic machine (exercise is discussed in Chapter 5);
- following a high-fibre diet with plenty of fruit, vegetables, whole grain, pulses, nuts and seeds (diet is discussed in Chapter 6).

If you suffer from venous ulcers, your vascular surgeon will recommend surgical treatment for your varicose veins. This should help the ulcers to heal and protect against further ulcers forming (see Chapters 8 and 9).

Vein rupture

When a varicose vein ruptures and starts to bleed, the amount of blood loss can be alarming. In the past, people have even died from severe blood loss related to a varicose rupture, usually because they didn't know how to stem the flow. It is fortunate that bleeding is a rare complication, and it can occur only when the skin covering the varicose veins is thin and damaged and the affected vein is very prominent – usually in the lower leg.

However, you don't need to knock or bump your leg to experience a varicose vein bleed – it can happen spontaneously. If, for whatever reason, it does start to bleed, lie down with your leg propped up on cushions, a stool or a chair, then apply pressure to the bleeding area. Using a tourniquet can make matters worse, so use a clean cloth of some kind and press it hard to the area for about 15 minutes. The bleeding can always be controlled in this way because the pressure of blood in the veins is low. (If an artery had begun bleeding, it would be a different story entirely, for arterial bleeds are difficult to stem. Fortunately, varicosities do not develop in arteries.)

When the bleeding has stopped, place a clean pad to the area and firmly wrap a bandage around it. You should now visit your doctor or local accident and emergency department immediately. Not only is a bleeding varicose vein a potential medical emergency, but plans need to be made for surgical intervention to avoid repeats of the incident (see Chapters 8 and 9 for information about treatments).

Theories behind the mechanism of skin damage and ulceration

Despite considerable research into varicose skin damage, there is still a lot that we don't know. Unfortunately, once the tissues have become damaged, they will never return to normal and may always be prone to poor healing and ulceration. You can improve the situation, however, by treating the underlying venous problems and using good-quality compression stockings. Compression stockings will also stop the problem from worsening.

The fibrin cuff theory

One of the substances that promote the clotting of blood is called *fibrin*, which has been shown in microscopic examination of damaged skin to produce a 'cuff' around the capillaries. Previously, this cuff was believed to restrict the flow of oxygen from the blood to the tissues. Recent research, however, has indicated that this is not the principal cause of damage to the skin and fatty layer beneath it.

The trapping of white blood cells theory

Research on damaged capillaries at the ankle has shown that white blood cells – also called *leucocytes* – become trapped when pressure in the veins is high. White blood cells contain a potent mixture of substances that produce inflammation when stimulated to do so. After sticking to certain receptors on the capillary walls, they discharge inflammatory substances that are thought to damage the tissues over a long period.

Rather than seeing the fibrin cuff as the cause of skin and fat damage, researchers are now theorizing that chronic inflammation is the culprit – caused by white blood cells being trapped over a long period of time.

4

Pregnancy and the veins

During pregnancy, hormonal changes and an increased volume of blood affect the walls of the veins and predispose the woman to numerous vein problems, from varicose veins, pelvic congestion syndrome and phlebitis to deep vein thrombosis (known as DVT).

Varicose veins in pregnancy

Throughout the 9 months of pregnancy, it is fairly common for varicose veins to appear spontaneously and for any existing varicose veins to enlarge. Such varicose veins normally arise in the calf and thigh areas, but in some cases surprisingly large ones can appear in the vulva and vaginal walls. Varicose veins in the female genital area are prone to being painful. This not only creates problems for walking, sitting and doing the things that are part of normal life, it also makes sexual intercourse difficult and, for many women, embarrassing.

Some fortunate women carry several children without ever a sign of a varicose vein. However, there are plenty of others who develop them early in their first pregnancy, others who develop them further on in the first pregnancy, and yet others who don't develop them until their second, third or fourth pregnancy. Often, the swollen veins disappear shortly after the baby is born, but there is less likelihood of this with each subsequent pregnancy. Indeed, varicose veins tend to worsen with each pregnancy and are likely to enlarge throughout the 9 months.

Varicose veins are usually harmless in the short term. Your doctor will want you to wait until your pregnancy is over before treatment is considered – that is if they are still in existence then.

Who gets varicose veins during pregnancy?

Women are more likely to develop varicose veins during pregnancy if:

- other family members have them;
- they are carrying twins or higher multiples, because this adds to the pressure of blood in the legs, and so makes them more prone;
- they are overweight;
- they stand for long periods.

Why varicose veins develop during pregnancy

There are several reasons why varicose veins can appear or worsen in pregnancy:

- The growing uterus exerts increasing pressure on the vena cava (the large vein on the right side of the body that drains the legs), and this increase in pressure in turn increases the pressure of blood in the leg veins – veins that already have to work against gravity to return blood to the heart.
- The volume of blood in the body increases during pregnancy, overburdening the valves that push the blood in the legs upwards.
- There are raised levels of the hormone progesterone in pregnancy, and progesterone has the effect of causing blood vessels to relax and stretch.

Blood clots in pregnancy

During pregnancy, tiny blood clots in the superficial veins near the surface of the skin can develop in a small percentage of women. This causes the vein to feel rope-like and hard, and the area around it may be hot, red, tender or painful.

Although blood clots in the superficial veins are seldom serious, you should visit your doctor if you think you have one. It is possible for the area around the clot to become infected, causing a high temperature, chills and, often, a headache. Antibiotic medication is the best treatment for this. You should also see your doctor without delay if your legs or ankles swell significantly, if sores break out or the skin near the veins changes colour.

Genetic tendency to blood clots

Researchers have found a genetic tendency to developing blood clots and that women carrying the *factor V Leiden* gene have a substantially increased risk of clotting in pregnancy (and also when they are taking oestrogen-based birth control pills or hormone replacement therapy (HRT)). Women with this gene also have a greater chance of developing pre-eclampsia – a state in pregnancy in which the blood pressure is raised and there is protein in the urine. Pre-eclampsia ensures that the woman is confined to hospital for the remainder of her pregnancy. To reduce the risk of the more dangerous eclampsia occurring – in which the woman can suffer seizures and maybe even die – her labour may be induced early.

Factor V Leiden has also been found to be a contributing factor in miscarriage and stillbirth due to clotting in the placenta, umbilical cord or the foetus itself, although clotting will occur in the foetus only if the baby has inherited the gene.

The reason that some women with factor V Leiden experience clots and others don't is believed to be due largely to nutritional and lifestyle factors. If you are pregnant, or planning to get pregnant, following the advice in this book can make a great difference to the outcome.

Deep vein thrombosis

The vast majority of people with the above-mentioned gene are unaware that they have it. It may only be diagnosed after repeated miscarriage or the development of clots within weeks of becoming pregnant. Serious deep vein thrombosis (DVT) is a very real, but rare, complication of this condition – approximately one in 1,000 women experience it during pregnancy or in the weeks after delivery. Women on bed rest or who have blood clotting disorders are at higher risk, however. The warning signs of DVT are sudden tenderness and swelling, and pain that does not subside, as well as features of pulmonary embolism (shortness of breath with pain, localized pain that does not subside and a 'bruised' feeling on inhaling).

If DVT is diagnosed, you will be hospitalized immediately and treated with injections of a blood-thinning agent for the remainder of the pregnancy and for 4–6 weeks after the baby is delivered.

During pregnancy, a drug such as enoxaparin sodium that does not cross over to the baby and cause birth defects will be used – which rules out warfarin. However, warfarin can be used after pregnancy because it does not cross over into breast milk.

If DVT is not treated, there is a chance of a pulmonary embolism occurring (when a blood clot breaks away and travels through the veins to the lungs). The symptoms of a pulmonary embolism include coughing (maybe coughing up blood), shortness of breath, painful breathing, a rapid heartbeat and a feeling of panic. An untreated pulmonary embolism can lead to death.

A person who experiences a DVT during pregnancy stands a higher chance of it returning during any subsequent pregnancies. Therefore, in such cases, preventative treatment is likely to be offered.

Phlebitis in pregnancy

In a woman who is prone to developing varicose veins, there is a greater risk of phlebitis occurring during pregnancy. Phlebitis is inflammation of the vein walls and it presents as a reddened lumpiness or a red line under the skin at the site of a previous varicose vein. The condition usually resolves itself with time, elevation (see Chapter 5) and a course of non-steroidal anti-inflammatory drugs. Depending on the degree of inflammation, antibiotics may also be prescribed. If episodes of phlebitis persist during the course of the pregnancy, you are likely to be referred for Doppler ultrasound examination of the deep veins to ensure that there is no underlying DVT. If this test is not offered, ask your doctor why not.

Pelvic congestion syndrome

An estimated one third of all women experience chronic pelvic pain at some time in their lives. Until recently, doctors believed it was a phantom pain – that is, 'all in the mind'. However, recent advances have shown that it can result from varicose veins in the pelvic region – a condition known as pelvic congestion syndrome (PCS).

The condition is caused by the same sequence of events that makes varicose veins develop in the legs – the valves that help to return blood to the heart become weakened and don't close properly, allowing blood to pool in the area and the veins to bulge. It is estimated that up to 15 per cent of women have varicose veins in the pelvic region, but not all of them experience symptoms.

The risk factors for the onset of PCS are:

- pregnancy;
- an increase in hormone levels from taking the contraceptive pill or HRT;
- varicose veins, or full leg veins;
- polycystic ovaries;
- hormonal dysfunction.

Because women lie down for a pelvic examination, which takes pressure off the varicosities, PCS is difficult for doctors to detect. Many women with this syndrome spend years trying to find out what's wrong with them – and living with an undiagnosed chronic condition affects not only the woman, but also her interactions with her family and friends and her general outlook on life. There is treatment for PCS, but in the absence of a diagnosis, this will not be offered.

The symptoms arising with PCS include a dull, aching pain in the lower abdomen and lower back. The pain normally increases during a woman's menstrual periods, when she is tired, when she is standing, during pregnancy and following sexual intercourse. There can also be vaginal discharge, excessive menstrual bleeding, an irritable bladder, and varicosities on the vulva, buttocks or thigh areas.

If you are diagnosed with PCS, you can take over-the-counter naproxen sodium or ibuprofen to alleviate the symptoms. Where there is not significant improvement, you are likely to be referred to a gynaecologist to discuss further treatment options. In the event that your doctor is unable or unwilling to diagnose the cause of your chronic pelvic pain, don't hesitate to get a second opinion. It is essential that you are examined thoroughly, too, to ensure that nothing more serious is wrong.

Prevention and treatment of varicose veins in pregnancy

A woman who didn't have varicose veins before she got pregnant is far more likely to see improvements after birth than a woman who already had varicose veins. Whether or not you have experienced varicose veins in the past, the following advice can help to prevent them, or minimize their effects:

- Take daily exercise to boost your circulation. A brisk 10-minute walk is better than nothing – but aim for 20 minutes.
- Try to keep within the recommended weight range for your stage of pregnancy.
- Try to raise your feet and legs whenever you are resting. Prop up the bottom of your bed with blocks or books.
- When sitting, avoid crossing your legs, or even your ankles.
- Avoid standing still for long periods. Take plenty of strolls around.
- Try to spend most of the night on your left side and tilt yourself slightly to the left when you are sitting. As the inferior vena cava vein is located on the right side, lying on your left or leaning to the left lessens the weight of the uterus on the vein. This reduces pressure on the veins in your legs and feet.
- Wear good support stockings.

5

Self-help measures

Making certain lifestyle changes can – as discussed in this chapter – prevent varicose veins from occurring and limit the symptoms if they already exist. Such changes can also help to stop their spread.

Exercise

Because it boosts circulation, improves muscle tone and strengthens the vein walls, exercise is an important component of any health-related self-help programme. When the calf muscles are exercised, they act as a pump (this is the 'muscle pump', as mentioned earlier), taking over the job that weak valves have become less capable of doing. Therefore, the stronger your calf muscles and the more you move them, the better your circulation. The muscle pump is always encouraged into action by exercise. Moreover, staying fit is the best way to keep your leg muscles toned and your weight under control.

It is recommended that you try to carry out an exercise regime daily, focusing on exercises that work your legs. If, for any reason, you are unable to follow the exercises given in this chapter, ask your doctor to refer you to an exercise therapist who is knowledge-able about the particular needs of the condition. You will then be taught a programme of exercise to suit your needs.

Warm-ups

It is important to warm up and mobilize the muscles and joints before embarking on any aerobic and weight-bearing exercise. Warm-ups increase your body temperature and the flow of blood to the working areas, preparing the cardiovascular system for exertion. Warm-ups also help to prevent muscular soreness and injury. Never skip warm-ups in favour of more vigorous exercise.

Stand with your feet about 40cm (15 inches) apart, keep your body relaxed, your back straight, your bottom tucked in and your stomach flattened as you perform your routine. All exercises should be smooth and continuous. If you don't have full movement in any joint, stretch it as far as you can without causing discomfort. You should find that you gain more and more flexibility as you repeat the exercise on a long-term basis.

I have included exercises for other areas of your body to help warm up your whole system:

- Neck: slowly turn your head to the left then hold to a count of two. Return to the centre and repeat the exercise 10 times. Now turn your head to the right then hold to a count of two before returning to the centre. Repeat 10 times. Tucking in your chin a little, tilt your head down and hold to a count of two before returning to the centre. Repeat 10 times. Finally, tilt your head upwards and hold to a count of two before returning to the centre. Repeat 10 times.
- Spine (first set of warm-ups): placing your hands on your hips to help support your lower back, slowly tilt your upper body to the left and hold to a count of two. Return to the centre, and repeat between 2 and 10 times. Now tilt to the right and return to the centre. Repeat between 2 and 10 times.
- Spine (second set of warm-ups): keeping your lower back static, swing your arms and upper body to the left as far as they will comfortably go, then return to the centre. Repeat 10 times. Now swing your arms and upper body to the right and return to the centre. Repeat 10 times.
- Hips and knees: with your body upright, move your hips by lifting your left knee upwards, as far as is comfortable. Hold to a count of two, then lower. Now raise your right knee and hold to a count of two. Repeat 10 times.
- Ankles: with your supporting leg bent slightly, place your left toes on the floor in front of you. Lift up your foot and then place your left heel on the floor. Repeat 10 times. Now duplicate the exercise with the right foot.

Pulse-raising activities

Pulse-raising activities, another part of your warm-up routine, should build up gradually. Their purpose is to warm your muscles further in preparation for stretching. Marching on the spot for 2–4 minutes: starting slowly, then speeding up a little more is ideal. If you aren't able to spend so long marching on the spot, do as much as you can, building up slowly. Remember that every little helps!

Stretching exercises

Stretches prepare the muscles for the more challenging movements to follow, if you are up to them:

- Calf (first set of stretching exercises): stand with your arms out-stretched and your palms against a wall. Keeping your left foot on the floor, bend your left knee. Press the heel of your right foot into the floor until you feel a gentle stretch in your leg muscles. Now change legs, alternating between the left and right leg. Repeat 10 times.
- Calf (second set of stretching exercises): standing with your feet slightly apart, raise both heels off the floor so that you are on your toes. Repeat 10 times. As your calf muscles strengthen you should be able to stay on your toes for longer periods of time.
- Front of thigh: using a chair or the wall for support, stand with your left leg in front of your right, both knees bent, your right heel off the floor. Tuck in your bottom, and move your hip forwards until you feel a gentle stretch in the front of your right thigh. Now alternate legs. Repeat 10 times.
- Back of thigh: stand with your legs slightly bent and your left leg about 20cm (8 inches) in front of your right leg. Keeping your back straight, place both hands on your hips and lean forward a little. Now straighten your left leg, tilting your bottom upwards until you feel a gentle stretch in the back of your left thigh. Now alternate legs. Repeat 10 times.
- Groin: spreading your legs slightly, your hips facing forward and your back straight, bend your left leg and move your right leg slowly sideways until you feel a gentle stretch in your groin. Gently move to the right, bending your right leg as you straighten the left.

Aerobic exercise

Aerobic exercise – an activity that makes you slightly out of breath – should come next. This type of exercise aids overall fitness and encourages weight loss in those who are overweight. Try to choose an activity that you will enjoy and will want to continue.

People with varicose veins require moderate exercise instead of more strenuous activity (such as jogging, high-impact aerobics, strenuous cycling or any activity that increases the blood pressure in the veins). Instead, low-impact activities are recommended, such as walking, swimming, low-impact aerobics and moderate weight training.

If you are pregnant, it is not wise to raise your body's core temperature. Stick to the warm-ups and stretching exercises. Note that, whether or not you are pregnant, you should check with your doctor before embarking on regular aerobic activity:

- Walking: this most convenient low-impact aerobic activity aids mobility, strength and stamina, and helps to protect against osteoporosis. You may find it easier to use a treadmill, reading a book or magazine at the same time or listening to a personal music player, the radio or audio (story) tapes. Aim to walk for 20 or 30 minutes at a time. A treadmill should never wholly replace outdoor walking.
- Stepping: start with a fairly small step (for example, a wide, hefty book, such as a catalogue or a telephone directory), or, if you wish, use a step machine or the bottom step of your staircase. Place first your left foot, then your right foot on to the book or step. Now step backwards, first with your left foot, then with your right. Repeat for 2–10 minutes, then change feet, placing first your right foot on the step, then your left.
- Trampoline jogging: jogging on a small, circular trampoline can provide a good aerobic work-out. If you can manage to get into a rhythm, the trampoline will do much of the work for you. Try to jog in this way for 20–30 minutes. Small, inexpensive trampolines are available from most exercise equipment outlets.
- Cycling: whether you use a stationary or ordinary bicycle, this form of activity provides an efficient cardiovascular work-out. It is best to start by pedalling slowly and gradually building up

momentum – and at first limit your sessions to 2 or 3 minutes, building up to 15 or 20 minutes, if possible. Avoid doing strenuous cycling, however, as the pressure build-up of blood in the pelvis can actually cause varicose veins.

Strength and endurance exercises

If you feel you have done enough at this point, run through the cool-down exercises then congratulate yourself for doing something positive to help yourself. Perhaps when you feel fitter you can incorporate this section into your routine. Again I have included exercises for other areas of your body to improve your circulation and general health – it's up to you whether you carry them out:

- Thighs (first set of strength and endurance exercises): lean back against a wall with your feet 30cm (12 inches) away from the base of the wall. With your posture aligned, slowly squat down, keeping your heels on the ground. Now slowly straighten your legs again. Repeat between 2 and 10 times.
- Thighs (second set of strength and endurance exercises): holding on to a sturdy chair and keeping your back 'tall', bend and then slowly straighten both legs, keeping your heels on the floor. Repeat the exercise between 2 and 10 times.
- Upper back: lie face down on the floor and, keeping your legs straight, gently raise your head and shoulders. Hold to a count of two, then lower them. Repeat between 2 and 10 times.
- Lower back: lie on your back and lift your right leg, pulling it towards your chest until you feel a gentle pull in your bottom and lower back. Repeat with the left leg. Now pull both legs up together. Repeat each exercise between 2 and 10 times.
- Abdomen: lie on your back with your knees bent and your feet flat on the floor. Now raise your head and shoulders, reaching with your arms towards your knees. Remember to keep the middle of your back on the floor.
- Push-ups: stand with your hands flat against a wall, your body straight. Carefully lower your body towards the wall, then slowly push away. Repeat 2 to 10 times.

Exercise while you sit

If you are in a situation where you are unable to get up and walk around – in an office meeting or on an aeroplane flight, for example, it is important to do simple exercises to keep the blood pumping through your legs. About once every half hour, lift your toes while keeping your heels down, as though you are pumping a piano pedal. Repeat for a couple of minutes. Now lift your heels while keeping your toes down and repeat for a couple of minutes.

Compression

Compression stockings are often prescribed by doctors for patients with more severe varicose veins. They are elastic stockings that are made to fit the dimensions of your leg, not the size of your foot. They squeeze the leg veins to stop excess blood flowing backwards, thereby decreasing the severity of symptoms. As a result, the following advantages are gained:

- there is less pooling of blood in the affected veins;
- blood flow within the affected veins is increased;
- the muscle pump becomes more efficient;
- sores are encouraged to heal and prevented from returning;
- there is usually an improvement in the way fluid is filtered from the tissues into the capillaries, and when prolonged swelling is present, good compression can reduce it and make it less likely to recur.

In milder cases, wearing ordinary support stockings or tights may offer sufficient benefit. They are available from most high-street chemists and provide support all the way up the leg. For more serious varicose veins, there are specially made graduated stockings or bandages that are available on prescription from your doctor or for purchase at surgical appliance shops and certain chemists. 'Graduated' compression means that the compression is greatest at the ankle and that the stockings become gradually less tight further up the leg. Such stockings may need to be worn daily for the rest of your life and may be all that is required to relieve pain and swelling and to prevent future problems. A key is to take your bath or shower at night rather than in a morning. As soon as you get out of bed in the morning, pull on the stockings before your veins have the chance to become more swollen. If you find, on trying compression stockings, that your pain and discomfort worsens, especially after walking, take them off immediately and ask your doctor's advice. There may be a problem with the blood supply to your legs – that is, the arterial blood supply that carries oxygen to your tissues.

Graduated compression stockings are usually a pale brown 'skin' colour, but they do come in black and other 'skin' shades. They are available in below-knee length and above-knee length. Below-knee length stockings are usually more comfortable to wear than above-knee stockings, and they are suitable for people with ankle swelling and problems in the lower part of the limb. People with varicosities above the knees need to use above-knee stockings, held up by suspenders or a special belt. Unfortunately, this type of stocking is a source of embarrassment for many users, particularly men.

Compression stockings come in different strengths, or classes:

- Class 1 – this type of stocking contains the lowest level of compression. However, for most people, it is sufficient to relieve the symptoms of varicose veins.
- Class 2 – this type of stocking is stronger, providing good support for varicose veins. Its strength is sufficient to aid the prevention of leg swelling, skin damage (lipodermatosclerosis) and ulceration. It may be most useful for patients of a slim build, with slim legs.
- Class 3 – this type of stocking is the strongest available and recommended for people with skin damage, leg swelling that has not been controlled by class 2 stockings and a tendency for developing ulcers. It may be most useful for patients with large, heavy legs.

Because some people have very thick or unusually shaped legs, the circumference of the leg must be measured at a few levels before the one with the best fit can be selected. It is important that your stockings are a good fit and feel comfortable because, unfortunately, you may have to wear them for the rest of your life. If the stockings that are available do not fit properly or are not sufficiently long, it is possible to have stockings custom-made. Ask your doctor about this.

If you find your compression stockings difficult to put on, as many people do, don't be afraid to ask for help from your partner or a friend. If this is not possible, there are now tools, which your doctor can tell you about, that can make the task much easier. Compression stockings are often found to be uncomfortable, especially in hot weather, but no advantage will be gained from wearing them rolled down.

In some cases, elevation, exercise and the use of compression stockings will fail to improve the condition of your varicose veins and you may require a surgical treatment. Surgical procedures are discussed in Chapters 8 and 9. A word of warning: try not to fall into the habit of sitting with your feet up for most of the day. If you are wearing good compression stockings, make an effort to remain as active as you can.

Four-layer bandaging

Venous ulcers have been shown to respond best to a 'four-layer bandage' system, applied by a specially trained nurse. There is a slight risk of skin damage, however, in people with restricted arterial blood flow. It is therefore important to have your leg arteries checked before this system is used.

Care of stockings

Owing to daily wear and regular washing, compression stockings lose some of their elasticity over time. It is important, therefore, that they are replaced every 3–4 months. Older stockings will fail to do their job.

Elevation of the legs

Standing for long periods and sitting for hours with your feet on the ground or with your legs crossed are sure-fire ways of bringing on symptoms from your varicose veins. However, you can prevent symptoms from worsening by putting your legs up, which helps to decrease the pressure in the veins of the leg. To obtain maximum effect, elevate your legs above the level of your heart for 15–30 minutes at intervals throughout the day. If it's not always possible for you to raise your legs above your heart, place your feet on a level with your body. Putting them on a low stool, or the other end of the sofa is not enough. Also, do not sit with your legs crossed at all, either at the knees or ankles.

If you are required to stand or sit (with your feet on the ground) for prolonged periods – such as on a long car journey or in the office – it's recommended that you walk around once every hour to allow the muscles to pump the blood out of the veins. As mentioned earlier, it's not easy to get up in some situations, so you should try to go up and down on your toes frequently, raising and lowering your heels. This is not ideal, but it does help to pump blood upwards and reduces the constant pressure on your legs.

A great exercise to drain blood from swollen veins is to lie flat on the floor and rest your legs on the seat of a chair or straight up against a wall for 2 minutes. Using a recliner chair can also help the blood to flow back to the heart from the legs, but remember not to recline in it for too long at a time.

Tilting the bed

A simple remedy for varicose veins is to place bricks, books or blocks of wood under the footboard of your bed so that your feet are raised a few centimetres while you are sleeping. This discourages the blood from pooling in your limbs and helps the muscle pump to work.

If you have a history of heart problems or difficulty breathing during the night – including sleep apnoea – you should consult your doctor before tilting your bed in this way.

Clothing

Many people unwittingly restrict their circulation by wearing clothing that is too tight. As a result, blood is not able to flow through the body as it should and varicose veins are made even more problematic. Some experts believe that constantly wearing tight clothing can even cause varicose veins. Clothing such as snug-fitting girdles or corsets, skin-tight trousers, tights, pop-socks, socks with tight elastic tops, tight belts, some boots and shoes (especially high heels) can cut off the circulation and either force the blood to search out an alternative route, maybe even through the deep veins, or cause back-pressure on the veins. Over time, the extra blood causes the veins to weaken and stretch, resulting in varicose veins.

Try as many self-help measures as you like, but nothing much will change until you stop wearing tight clothing and high heels.

Self-help recommendations

Below are the recommendations for the prevention and treatment of varicose veins. Most topics have already been mentioned, but there is some additional advice:

- Follow a daily exercise regime to stay fit and boost your circulation.
- Take a brisk walk every day – 10 minutes is better than nothing, but aim for 20 minutes.
- Try to keep your weight within the average range for your height and build.
- Try to raise your feet and legs whenever you are resting. Prop up the footboard of your bed.
- When sitting, avoid crossing your legs and ankles.
- Avoid standing still for long periods. Take plenty of short strolls.
- Sleep mostly on your left side.
- Wear good support stockings.
- Avoid wearing tight clothing and, for women, high heels.
- Drink plenty of water.
- If your doctor agrees, take aspirin or ibuprofen tablets when the pain is bad.
- If you smoke, try to stop. Smoking can contribute to raised blood pressure and so exacerbate varicose veins.
- Follow a healthy balanced diet, as discussed in Chapter 6.

6

A nutritional approach to varicose veins

It is widely accepted that a healthy balanced diet that is high in fruits, vegetables and whole grain and low in fat and refined carbohydrates is capable of improving many health conditions. Where varicose veins are concerned, a good diet cannot only improve your overall health, it can also reduce the pressure in the affected leg or legs and eliminate constipation – straining can cause and worsen varicose veins (see below).

The recommended diet for the prevention and treatment of varicose veins is as described in this chapter. There should be emphasis, however, on the following:

- fresh fruits, including berries and cherries;
- citrus fruits – and don't forget to nibble on the inside of the rind, which is a useful source of helpful nutrients;
- whole grains;
- garlic;
- onions;
- ginger;
- cayenne pepper.

Curing constipation

Constipation is believed to be one of the leading causes of varicose veins. Straining to pass a stool on the toilet can greatly restrict blood flow as it returns to the torso through the deep veins in the legs. The blood backs up and finds an outlet down the superficial veins, where it can pool and form bulging varicosities. However, as mentioned earlier, a high-fibre diet is likely to relieve constipation and eliminate the need to strain. If changing your diet doesn't help, ask your doctor's advice. You may need to take a fibre supplement on a regular basis.

There is no doubt that consuming a lot of fibre is good for us. Formerly known as roughage, fibre is the indigestible part of plants, the cellulose fibre that forms the leaf webbing in green vegetables, the skins of sweetcorn and beans, and the husks of wheat and corn. It is found in fruits, vegetables, nuts, seeds, beans, peas, lentils, wholemeal breads and cereals (wheat, oats, rye, barley, quinoa, spelt, buckwheat, corn etc).

Fibre is useful to us all not only because of its high nutritional content, but also because it is a bulking agent that quickly sweeps the bowel clean, ensuring that no unhealthy waste products lurk in hidden corners. It is recommended that you consume at least 30g of fibre a day. To achieve this, you will need to build your meals around fruits and vegetables, whole grains and legumes, which are discussed below. In addition, try to eat plenty of cherries, blueberries (bilberries) and blackberries – they contain important compounds that can prevent varicose veins or lessen their symptoms.

Some experts recommend going on a juice diet one day a week to encourage regularity. See page 65 for information on 'juice therapy'.

Losing excess weight

If you are overweight, you are unwittingly exerting unnecessary pressure on your legs, causing your varicose vein symptoms to be worse than they need be. It also creates extra pressure on your heart and circulatory system. Therefore, your best course of action is to lose weight – which is easier said than done. You don't have to go hungry to shed the kilos, however – you need only to eat a balanced whole-food diet, as described below.

If a surgical procedure is seen as the only real option for your varicose vein problems, your surgeon might ask you to lose weight beforehand. This is because post-operative wound infection and deep vein thrombosis are more likely in overweight people. Also, there is a greater chance of varicose veins recurring in a person who is overweight.

A balanced whole-food diet

Whole-foods are simply those that have had nothing taken away – that is, they still contain nutrients and fibre – and that have had nothing added – that is, no colourings, flavourings, preservatives and so on have been added. In short, whole-foods are foods in their most natural form. If you can ensure that many of the foods you eat are as close to their original state as possible, you will be doing yourself a great service. You may prefer to cook most of your vegetables, but do try to eat them raw when you can – raw onion and grated raw carrots are tasty with a salad, and raw carrot and cabbage are part of a coleslaw. Don't forget that every little helps!

The other components of the recommended diet are discussed below.

Fresh fruits and vegetables

Fresh fruits and vegetables are an essential part of any healthy diet. They contain fibre as well as many important vitamins, minerals and enzymes. Try to eat them as fresh and as raw as possible. Make a variety of salads and try to eat a salad every day. When you do cook vegetables, boil them in unsalted (or lightly salted) water for the minimum length of time. Lightly steaming and stir-frying are healthy alternatives. Scrub rather than peel your vegetables.

It is recommended that people with varicose veins consume blackberries, blueberries (bilberries) and cherries on a regular basis. These fruits contain compounds that support the normal formation of connective tissue (collagen) and that strengthen the veins and capillaries. As such, they can help to prevent or treat varicose veins.

Legumes (peas and beans)

Legumes are high in protein and usually inexpensive to buy. The soya bean is a complete protein, meaning that it contains all the amino acids that human beings require. There are many soya bean products, including soya milk, tofu, tempeh and miso. Tofu, for example, is very versatile and can be used in both savoury and sweet dishes.

Seeds

Sunflower, sesame, hemp and pumpkin seeds contain a wonderful combination of nutrients – all necessary to start a new plant – and are important to good health. They can be eaten as they are as a snack, sprinkled on to salads and cereals, or used in baking. For more flavour they can be lightly roasted and coated with organic soy sauce.

Nuts

Nuts, too, are an intrinsic part of any healthy diet. All nuts contain vital nutrients, but almonds, cashews, walnuts, Brazil nuts and pecans offer the greatest array. Eat a wide assortment as snacks, with cereal and in baked foods.

Grains

Whole grains and wholemeal flours provide us with the complex unrefined carbohydrates that our bodies require – and organic is best. Aim to consume a variety of grains, including oats, rye, barley (generally available as pearl barley), corn, buckwheat, brown rice and mixed grains. Oats are highly recommended, too, as they help to stabilize blood sugar levels.

Fish

Try to eat plenty of fish, especially the oily fish such as sardines, tuna, mackerel, trout, salmon, herring, pilchards and kippers. Cut down on red meat as much as possible. When you do eat red meat, make sure it is no larger or thicker than the palm of your hand.

Garlic, onions, ginger and cayenne pepper

As these foods are all highly recommended for the prevention and treatment of varicose veins. Try to eat them as often as you can.

Reducing salt

Although our bodies need a certain amount of the sodium that we obtain from salt, a high intake can be harmful in many ways. High blood pressure and heart disease are only two conditions that are linked to high salt consumption. Where varicose veins are concerned, more than a moderate salt consumption can cause water retention, which in turn can give rise to swelling in the lower leg and ankle. Such swelling results in increased pressure on the veins, and further varicosities.

If you have a propensity towards swelling, try to restrict the amount of salt you eat.

Salt as a preservative

Owing to its ability to inhibit the growth of harmful micro-organisms, high levels of salt are added as a preservative to most processed and pre-packaged foods. For example, one tin of soup contains more salt (sodium) than the recommended daily allowance for an adult. Large amounts of salt are also added to most breakfast cereals, except for shredded wheat products.

It is recommended, therefore, that you limit your intake of salt in the following ways:

- reduce your consumption of processed and pre-packaged foods;
- when you must buy processed and pre-packaged foods, look for 'low-salt' or 'sodium-free' on the label;
- use only a very small amount of salt (preferably sea salt or rock salt) in baking and cooking;
- try to avoid sprinkling any type of salt over your meals.

Reducing your salt intake very gradually is the best way to retrain your palate.

Reducing stimulants

One of the main reasons we crave stimulants such as caffeine and cigarettes is high levels of stress. When we are stressed our bodies demand a boost of energy – a 'lift'. However, the lift that we obtain from stimulants is short-lived, unlike the damage that stimulants can cause to our bodies.

Cutting out stimulants can significantly raise energy levels; it can reduce anxiety and greatly improve the health of our nerve cells. If you find you are unable to completely eliminate stimulants from your diet, reduce them as much as possible – it *will* make a difference.

Sugar

You may be surprised to hear that sugar consumption has been linked with many disorders, from diabetes to heart disease and cancer. However, we do need a certain amount of sugar for conversion to energy. What you may not know is that we can actually obtain all the sugar we need from fruit and complex (unrefined) carbohydrates (grains, lentils and so on), which convert into sugar in the body as nature intended.

If you really need to sweeten your food and drinks, alternatives to refined white sugar include raw honey, barley malt and fruit juice sweetener (fructose). Muscovado sugar and demerara sugar (both of which are also referred to as 'soft brown sugar') are formed during the early stages of the sugar refining process and so contain more nutrients than refined white sugar. All of the sweeteners mentioned here can be used in cooking and baking.

Artificial sweeteners

Refined sugar and simple carbohydrates are best avoided if you are trying to eat healthily, so many people wonder if they can they be replaced by a sugar substitute such as aspartame. The short answer is no, not if you really want to be healthy. Aspartame is an excitatory neurotransmitter that can have deleterious effects on the brain; as such it is best avoided.

Many people consume food and drinks containing aspartame in an attempt to lose weight. However, this artificial sweetener creates a craving for carbohydrates, which only causes weight gain. When they stop using aspartame – in diet sodas, for example – they generally lose weight.

Nancy Markle, an expert on multiple sclerosis, stated at a recent World Environment Conference that aspartame can be dangerous to diabetics, multiple sclerosis patients and people with Parkinson's disease. Neurosurgeon Dr Russell Blakelock states in his book entitled *Excitotoxins: The Taste that Kills*[1] that the ingredients of aspartame can over-stimulate the neurones of the brain, giving rise to dangerous symptoms. Furthermore, Dr H. J. Roberts, a diabetic specialist, has written a book entitled *Defense against Alzheimer's Disease*[2], in which he states that aspartame poisoning increases the risk of developing Alzheimer's disease.

The unrefined sugars found naturally in fruit and vegetables are safe and nutritious. They also take longer to digest, which avoids a sugar rush to the bloodstream and thus an excessive production of insulin. Fortunately, there are natural sweeteners such as stevia and xylitol that are perfectly safe and available from health food shops.

Fats and oils

Saturated fat and trans-fatty acids have a negative effect on the circulatory system. They increase blood levels of bad cholesterol, decrease levels of good cholesterol and can lead to atherosclerosis – a disease of the arteries characterized by deposits of fatty material on the artery walls. Atherosclerosis can lead to heart disease and stroke because it impedes normal blood flow through the arteries.

Varicose veins are very much a circulatory disorder and can therefore be improved by consuming a diet that is low in saturated fat and fairly high in unsaturated fat. The two distinct types of fat are:

- Saturated fat – the bad fat – which comes mainly from animal sources and is generally solid at room temperature. Although margarine was, for many years, believed to be a healthier choice than butter, nutritionists have now revised their opinion, for some of the fats in the margarine hydrogenation process are changed into trans-fatty acids, which the body metabolizes as if they were saturated fatty acids – the same as butter. Butter is a valuable source of oils and vitamin A, but should be used very sparingly. Margarine, on the other hand, is an artificial product containing many additives.

- Unsaturated fat – also called polyunsaturated or monounsaturated fat – which has a protective effect on the heart and other organs. Omega-3 and omega-6 oils occur naturally in oily fish (mackerel, herring, sardines, tuna and so on), nuts and seeds, and is usually liquid at room temperature. It is recommended that we all eat oily fish at least three times a week and cold-pressed oil (olive, rapeseed, safflower and sunflower oil) daily, for dressings and in cooking. Olive oil is better suited for cooking than other oils because it suffers less damage from heat.

Eggs

You're no doubt aware that eggs are high in cholesterol, which is a type of fat. However, they also contain lecithin, which is a superb biological detergent capable of breaking down fats so they can be utilized by the body. Lecithin also prevents the accumulation of too many acid or alkaline substances in the blood and encourages the transport of nutrients through the cell walls. Eggs should be soft boiled or poached as a hard yolk will bind the lecithin, rendering it useless as a fat detergent.

It is recommended that you eat two or three eggs a week.

Retraining your palate

In comparison with the average Western diet, which has, by the addition of chemical flavourings, saturated fat, sugar, salt and so on, evolved largely to please the taste buds, a healthy diet is based on foods in their more natural form. It is essential, therefore, that you *slowly* retrain your palate to accept different tastes. For this reason, it is advisable to cut back gradually on the amounts of sugar, salt and saturated fat that you consume. It takes only 28 days of eating a food regularly for it to become a habit.

Alcohol

As alcohol can cause the veins in your legs to dilate, it's advisable to limit your intake. Having a drink or two on special occasions should cause no additional problems, however.

Vitamins

It is known that consuming certain vitamins can reduce the symptoms of varicose veins. The most helpful vitamins are as described below.

Vitamin A (beta-carotene)

Consumption of sufficient vitamin A (in the form of beta-carotene) is vital to the health of all the bodily tissues. It improves the integrity of the skin and the strength of the vein walls, making them less likely to bulge. It also helps varicose ulcers to heal quickly and it accelerates the repairing of scars and skin damage. Food sources of vitamin A include yellow and orange fruits and vegetables such as carrots, sweet potatoes, apricots, cantaloupe, papaya, pumpkin, melon and mango. Vitamin A can also be found in dark, leafy vegetables such as spinach, Brussels sprouts, broccoli, cabbage and parsley.

Vitamin A supplementation is likely to be helpful in the treatment of varicose veins. However, it should not be taken in pregnancy.

B complex vitamins

The B vitamins are invaluable for the reduction of stress, regulation of the nervous system and the production of energy. Because they also help to maintain strong blood vessels, they can be used as a preventative measure for varicose veins or as a treatment to stop their progression. Unlike most other vitamins, the B vitamins are all interdependent, meaning they work best when consumed in combination with each other.

The B vitamins can be obtained from whole grains, lentils, seeds, leafy green vegetables, oily fish, avocados, prunes, apricots, mushrooms, dried fruit, eggs, lean meat and poultry. However, the B vitamins tend to be unstable, which makes them easily destroyed in food preparation and cooking. Furthermore, they are quickly flushed through the body, so they need to be put back on a daily basis. One daily comprehensive supplement tablet as well as one tablespoonful of brewer's yeast can help to maintain or restore good-quality blood vessels.

Vitamin C and bioflavonoids

Vitamin C is very much the anti-stress vitamin. It is also a great aid to circulation, promotes the healing of sores (and other skin problems such as ulcers and scarring), and helps to strengthen the vein walls to prevent dilatation of the veins. Unfortunately, this vitamin is quickly used up in the body, and its levels are reduced by smoking, alcohol consumption, surgery, trauma, stress, exposure to pollutants and the use of certain medications. Vitamin C food sources include citrus fruits, strawberries, blackcurrants, tomatoes, broccoli, Brussels sprouts, cabbage, green melons, potatoes and peppers (capsicum). As this vitamin is easily destroyed by heat and over-processing, it is recommended that vegetables be steamed for as little time as possible.

If you wish to use vitamin C supplementation for the prevention or treatment of varicose veins, you may find that it is combined with bioflavonoids. The latter compounds increase the effectiveness of vitamin C by preventing it from being used up in the body. In effect, bioflavonoids are able to greatly improve the body's ability to absorb and retain vitamin C. Without bioflavonoids, vitamin C is ineffective.

Bioflavonoid food sources are citrus fruits, apricots, blueberries (bilberries), cherries, rose-hips and buckwheat. The bioflavonoid quercetin is often combined with vitamin C and has, in research, shown promise in the treatment of varicose veins.

Vitamin E

This vitamin is essential for the good health of the circulatory system, and it reduces the susceptibility to varicose veins. People who already have varicosities find that food sources or dietary supplements of vitamin E relieve the symptoms and may even resolve the condition. Gently rubbing vitamin E squeezed from capsules on to localized irritation and varicose ulcers can ease the discomfort and encourage healing. However, because this vitamin has anti-thrombin properties, people who are taking the drug warfarin should consult their doctor before supplementing their diet with vitamin E.

Good food sources of vitamin E are fish, eggs, leafy green vegetables and oil, seed and grain derivatives – for example, wheatgerm, safflower, avocados, nuts, sunflower oil and seeds, pumpkin seeds, linseeds, almonds, Brazil nuts, cashews, pecans, whole grain cereals and breads, wheatgerm, asparagus, dried prunes and broccoli.

Because a small number of people with varicose veins have a condition called moderate coagulation factor deficiency – in which an excess of vitamin E can cause dangerous bleeding – ask your doctor for advice before you start taking vitamin E supplementation.

Minerals

Certain minerals are known to improve varicose veins.

Magnesium

Magnesium is important for the absorption of some other vitamins and minerals. Its benefit in varicose veins is that it works to relax the arteries and muscles in the legs, thereby making the muscle pump more efficient. Good sources of magnesium include whole grains, leafy green vegetables, nuts (especially almonds and cashews), seeds, legumes, soy products and vegetables (especially broccoli and sweet corn), bananas and apricots.

There are many good magnesium supplements. Follow the label dosage instructions.

Calcium

Calcium helps to stimulate the circulatory system, discouraging blood pooling and the sluggishness of flow. Sugars, pastries, soft drinks, alcoholic beverages, breads, cakes, biscuits and sweets leach calcium out of the body, and may therefore promote the formation of varicose veins. Dairy products are good sources of calcium, but they should be eaten sparingly because they are often high in fat. Fortunately, many other good sources of calcium exist, such as nuts, seeds, blackstrap molasses, legumes, oranges, leafy green vegetables and sardines. It is recommended that you also use products that are fortified with calcium such as cereals, orange juices and soy milk.

If you are unsure that your diet is providing sufficient calcium, you could try taking a calcium supplement.

Zinc

Zinc is important in preventing and treating varicose veins because it aids the healing process and helps collagen to form – collagen being the main structure in connective tissue, such as skin and vein walls. This mineral also helps to maintain the proper concentration of vitamin E in the blood. Zinc is generally low in Western-style foods, and the vegetarian diet is particularly deficient. Food sources include the herb liquorice, seafood, (lean) meats, eggs, liver, wheatgerm, pumpkin seeds, sunflower seeds and ginseng.

If you would like to take a supplement of this mineral, follow the label dosage instructions.

Other supplements and remedies

Various other supplements and remedies have been found to be useful in the treatment of varicose veins.

Bromelain

Bromelain is an enzyme that helps to activate an important compound – one that promotes the breakdown of fibrin. (Fibrin is a protein that is formed when blood starts to clot.) Therefore, bromelain intake can help to stop blood from clotting.

Bromelain is extracted from the pineapple plant and is available in supplement form. Follow the label dosage instructions.

Lecithin

In an adequate diet, lecithin is produced by the liver and is required daily by every cell in the body. Although no studies have been conducted to prove this, it is believed to break down fats, to lower cholesterol and to boost blood circulation, which are all excellent aids to varicose veins. A major source of lecithin is eggs (see page 59) – but for supplement form it is often extracted from soybean oil.

Supplements are available from health food shops.

Tissue salts

A man named Dr Schuessler first created a remedy called 'tissue salts' from very low homoeopathic preparations. There are twelve different types and they work gently on the physical structure of the body, building, repairing and maintaining health. Specifically, taking two tablets daily of calcium fluoride, morning and evening, can greatly improve the elasticity of the blood vessel walls.

Chlorophyll

This chemical is not very well known in the world of nutrition, but it is important in the world of biology and plants. All green plants contain chlorophyll, including the vegetables asparagus, bell peppers (capsicum), broccoli, Brussels sprouts, green cabbage, celery, collard greens, spinach, parsley, green olives and many others. Chlorophyll has a chemical structure similar to one of the structures within our blood cells, as a result of which it provides stronger blood and helps to revitalize the vascular system. It is also a rich source of vitamin K, which helps to prevent bleeding.

Chlorophyll is available as a nutritional supplement from health food shops. Follow the label dosage instructions.

Cayenne pepper

To reduce a flare-up of varicose vein symptoms and to improve the blood flow in your legs, take 1 teaspoon of cayenne pepper in a cup of hot water three times a day. This remedy is usually very effective, but benefits may take a few weeks to become apparent. As a maintenance dose when the flare-up is over, take 1 teaspoon in hot water once or twice a day.

Aspirin

Taking aspirin every day can thin the blood and make it circulate more easily through the veins. Aspirin can therefore relieve the pain of varicose veins. It is important, however, to speak to your doctor about the possibility of your taking aspirin – it is not good for people with certain problems of the digestive tract, for example. If your doctor is happy for you to take it, you will either be given a regular prescription or be told which strength of aspirin to buy.

Epsom salts

Your circulation can be stimulated by placing two tablespoonfuls of Epsom salts into a quart of water. Chill half of the liquid and heat the other half. Using a clean flannel, alternate 2-minute icy-cold soaks with 2-minute hot soaks, placing the flannel over the varicose veins.

Cod liver oil and honey

Rubbing a blend of cod liver oil and honey on to the affected area of the legs and covering the area with a bandage can also stimulate circulation. Leave the bandage on overnight.

Vitamin K cream

The regular application of vitamin K cream can strength the capillaries and reduce the symptoms of varicose veins. The cream can be purchased from health food shops.

Juice therapy

Drinking fresh fruit juices can significantly improve varicosities. Extract juice from dark-coloured fruits such as blueberries (bilberries), cherries and blackberries – these fruits contain pigments called anthocyanins and proanthocyanidins, which tone and strengthen the blood vessel walls. Pineapple contains bromelain (see page 63), an enzyme that helps to prevent blood from clotting.

Far higher concentrations of these nutrients are provided by drinking the juice than by merely eating the fruit. For maximum results, drink eight ounces of fresh berry, cherry or pineapple juice once or twice a day. If you like, you can add other juices such as apple, citrus fruit, beetroot, carrot or celery to create a variety of tastes.

Supplements containing anthocyanins, proanthocyanidins or bromelain may be taken, as an alternative to juice therapy.

If you suffer from constipation, some experts recommend drinking juices all day on one day a week to encourage regularity of bowel movements.

7

Diagnosing the problem

If you have visible varicose veins and believe they are making your legs ache and feel heavy, you should see your doctor. You should also seek your doctor's advice if:

- your varicose veins have become red, swollen, or very warm and tender to the touch;
- sores or a rash have appeared on your leg with the varicose veins, in the area near the ankle;
- there is swelling around the ankle or calf;
- you think there are circulation problems in your foot (or feet) – feet that are feeling cooler than usual, that have changed colour (to a bluish, reddish or paler shade) or that sometimes tingle and feel numb can indicate poor circulation in that area, as can slow healing of sores and wounds in the lower legs and feet.

Seeing your doctor

When you visit your doctor, the first thing he or she will do is ask a series of questions about your symptoms. Some people find it difficult to remember everything that's been happening to them when put on the spot, and so it might be useful to write it all down before setting off. It's advisable to take note of all the symptoms that you have experienced in the previous few months, even if you think they can't possibly be related to varicose veins – it is better to tell your doctor too much than too little. Many people fall into the trap of relating only what they think is relevant, and leave out something that is actually important in making the diagnosis. Indeed, it may be that another diagnosis entirely should be given, but because the doctor hears only the symptoms that would point to troublesome varicose veins, the real diagnosis is missed. It is not uncommon for leg problems to be attributed to varicose veins when there is quite a different underlying problem.

A history of DVT?

A person who has previously experienced DVT will be referred for further medical investigation before being offered treatment for their varicose veins – the deep veins may be damaged. Moreover, a history of DVT makes you more prone to developing DVT again during a surgical procedure.

It should first be established whether you did experience a true DVT – it is possible to misunderstand an earlier diagnosis of superficial thrombophlebitis. If you were given a special X-ray or scan of the veins, or if you were treated with warfarin or heparin, it's likely that you did have DVT. If you are really not sure, just ask your doctor to look back through your medical records.

General health questions

Your doctor is likely to ask questions about your general health, whether you smoke and whether you have allergies. He or she will refer to your medical records to see which medications you are currently taking. As mentioned earlier, taking the contraceptive pill or hormone replacement therapy (HRT) can have significant bearing on varicose veins.

Your general fitness levels and the amount of walking you do may also be of interest to your doctor, as may your diet and alcohol consumption. In addition, you will be asked whether you have any other problems with your legs, such as arthritis, and whether you have ever sustained a leg fracture or other serious leg injury.

The physical examination

In order to check the appearance of your legs, your doctor will ask you to stand up so that your legs are filled with blood and therefore the extent and size of your varicosities are more apparent. You may even be asked to stand on a platform that is placed in good light. Any swelling of the ankles will be looked for, as will signs of lipodermatosclerosis (in which there is damage to your skin; see pages 26–7).

If your doctor thinks that surgical intervention may help, you will be referred to a consultant vascular surgeon. The surgeon will help you to decide whether you should actually receive surgical treatment.

Goals of treatment

Your surgeon's goals of treatment are primarily to ease your symptoms on a long-term basis and to prevent any future complications. If you are concerned only with easing your symptoms in the short-term – maybe because of a fear of surgical interventions, for instance – you may opt to try the simple self-care measures as described in Chapter 5, together with a healthier nutritional approach, as described in Chapter 6. Try to remember that varicose veins cannot get better if they are left alone. In fact, they slowly worsen over time. If self-help measures prove ineffective, early intervention in the form of medical treatment can stop your symptoms from getting worse.

Getting back to goals ... an improved cosmetic appearance of varicose legs is not top of the list of your surgeon's goals for you, but surgeons do understand that varicosities cause embarrassment and are pleased to be able to help people to present themselves in a way that is more satisfactory. Surgery is not always offered when concerns are purely cosmetic, however.

To achieve all three of the aforementioned goals (to ease symptoms, to prevent complications and to improve appearance), the treatment you are offered may include permanent surgical removal of the affected veins.

Who gets treatment?

Until long-term studies show the true value – whether it be positive or negative – of surgery for varicose veins, surgeons must do their utmost to identify the patients who will gain most from such treatment.

There are currently no national guidelines with regard to who should receive varicose vein surgery under the National Health Service (NHS). The NHS does, however, give priority to patients with complications such as eczema and ulcers.

Doppler ultrasound scan

To check whether the valves in your legs are functioning normally, your surgeon or specialist vascular sonographer may perform a pain-free test called a 'Doppler ultrasound'. This is an important test because it indicates the patients who require more detailed examination, such as by use of a duplex ultrasound scanner (see below).

In Doppler ultrasound, a small hand-held probe with an ultrasound beam that changes its sound frequency when placed near to a moving object or substance is placed over the leg veins to listen to the blood flow near the surface of the skin – a gel-like substance having been applied to the skin first. The ultrasound signal can be shown on a computer screen and recorded for analysis. Obviously, if there is no movement of blood in the vein, the Doppler machine produces no sound. If blood is flowing, it shifts the Doppler frequency, and the machine makes a noise. Depending on the tone and character of the sound, information about blood flow in the leg is obtained.

Doppler ultrasound can determine the following:

- whether the long superficial vein (LSV) is incompetent, and at what level;
- whether there is any blood flowing back down the vein, behind the knee – a sign of incompetent valves. Reflux in this region may point to incompetence in the short saphenous vein (SSV) or even the deep veins;
- whether there are incompetent perforator veins;
- whether the arterial blood supply to the leg and foot is normal.

Duplex ultrasound scan

The 'colour-flow' duplex ultrasound scanner provides a similar but far more accurate test than the Doppler ultrasound scanner. It ought to be the standard technique for the evaluation of patients with venous disease of any type – however, many surgeons still use guesswork to assess the location of problem veins and base their operations on this. There is evidence that failing to perform a duplex ultrasound scan results in approximately one third of patients not getting the most suitable surgical procedure. It is therefore not surprising that varicose veins quickly reappear in many patients. When you are being evaluated by your surgeon, don't be afraid to ask for a duplex ultrasound scan.

The duplex scanner itself is larger than the Doppler scanner and uses two types of ultrasound – a colour-coded flow in addition to grey scale; hence the term 'duplex'. One type of ultrasound is reflected off different tissues in the body, producing moving pictures on a computer screen. (This is the same sort of ultrasound scan that is used during pregnancy.) The second type of ultrasound produced by the duplex scanner gives a more sophisticated image than the Doppler scanner. It is used in conjunction with a special technique, allowing Doppler signals to be received from any depth within the body. It can therefore show whether blood is flowing the wrong way in any particular vein.

Symptoms behind the knee

Duplex scanning is used for people who appear to have reflux behind the knee. Problems in this area are given priority treatment as, besides being a sign of reflux in the SSV, it can indicate incompetence in the main deep vein. Without this type of ultrasound scan, the person might receive treatment to the LSV only, when in fact the SSV is incompetent, too. Surgery to only one of the superficial veins means that the treated vein will become incompetent again. See page 8 for more information on reflux.

If duplex scanning detects a problem in the deep veins, you will be offered treatment as a matter of urgency.

When varicose veins return

When varicose veins come back after surgery to remove or seal them, duplex scanning can indicate incompetent veins in the groin that require treatment. There may also be a previously undetected length of LSV in the thigh that needs dealing with. Other leg veins under pressure from incompetent perforator veins may also be found by this method and sealed up or removed.

Contrast venography

Contrast venography was once the mainstay of investigation into the deep vein system. It involves injecting a type of dye ('radio-paque' contrast material) into a vein in the foot. Tourniquets are placed along the leg to close up the superficial veins and force the dye into the deep vein system, hence showing up any problems. Contrast venography has now largely been replaced by duplex ultrasound imaging. However, it continues to give a more detailed result when used in high-risk cases, such as in a person who has a pulmonary embolism but no leg symptoms.

Contrast varicography

Injecting contrast material into a varicose vein allows the venous system in that leg to be evaluated by X-ray. Contrast varicography used to be one of the principal diagnostic techniques, but it is only used today to determine the extent of the disease and to locate all identifiable reflux points, prior to surgery.

Plethysmography

Plethysmography describes a variety of tests on the legs to investigate blood flow through the veins. When thorough investigation of the leg veins is required – in a small number of complex cases – the arterial pulsation of blood through the calf is measured by plethysmography to assess the severity of venous disease.

8

Treatment

Because swollen and twisted veins are readily visible on physical examination, making a diagnosis of varicose veins is relatively easy. It is when medical investigation has ruled out an additional more serious condition that a vascular surgeon will decide whether your symptoms warrant the offer of surgical treatment. The surgeon will be more inclined to suggest surgery if you have tried compression stockings and other self-help measures without success. However, the next step, whatever it is, will be a joint decision between the vascular surgeon and yourself.

It's fairly safe to say that people who are experiencing swelling, bleeding, thrombophlebitis, ulceration or skin damage will be offered treatment, whether they have tried self-help measures or not.

If yours is not regarded as an urgent case, the type of treatment that you are offered may depend largely on your surgeon's personal preferences. Some surgeons favour traditional open surgery whereas others prefer to use newer, less invasive procedures. Open surgery for varicose veins has now been used for more than a century, and it probably carries slightly less risk of complications than the newer techniques. The complications attributed to open surgical treatment have the following very low averages:

- deep vein thrombosis: 0.15 per cent;
- pulmonary embolism: 0.06 per cent;
- wound complications including infection: 2.2 per cent.

According to vascular expert, Dr Alun H. Davies of the Imperial College, Charing Cross Hospital, London, the jury is still out on the best way to treat patients with venous incompetence. Indeed, the recurrence rates of different treatments have yet to be correctly compared over a significant period. Dr Davies believes that, in future, vascular surgeons need either to be able to offer all the treatments or be prepared to refer patients on to a specialist in another area of vascular treatment who can give the best result.

Note that bulging surface veins are frequently caused by underlying problem veins. The best results are seen when both surface and any underlying varicosities are treated. When presented with bulging surface veins, your doctor should use duplex ultrasound scanning (see Chapter 7) to penetrate further into the leg and evaluate other veins. Not until all the varicosities are identified should a treatment plan be drawn up.

Cosmetic removal of varicose veins

Some people are acutely embarrassed by their varicose veins and feel that, as long as they are in evidence, they are unable to enjoy their lives. Their veins may not be causing their legs to ache, itch and feel heavy; indeed, they may have none of the other problems related to varicose veins, but emotional distress can be just as difficult to live with as any physical problem – more so, for some. It is unfortunate, though, that this fact is not fully appreciated by all medical professionals and therefore the removal of varicose veins for cosmetic reasons is not always an option. It is hoped that, in time, cosmetic treatment will be available for everyone who wants it.

If your surgeon is willing to get rid of your veins for cosmetic reasons, you will be informed about the inconvenience and risks of surgery before you make your final decision.

Sclerotherapy

Sclerotherapy is a non-surgical procedure in which a solution is injected into the varicose veins to improve their appearance and eliminate symptoms.

Injection sclerotherapy

Injection sclerotherapy – sometimes called *compression sclerotherapy* – is often the treatment of choice for patients with less pronounced varicose veins. It is usually carried out by a specialist member of the surgical team. As no anaesthetic is required, the risks associated with many surgical procedures are greatly reduced, and there is usually no pain. The treatment is provided on a hospital out-patient basis, taking between 15 minutes and 1 hour to perform. It involves the patient lying on an examination couch and the leg being raised to empty the veins. A fine needle injects a liquid chemical into the affected vein, causing damage to the vein walls and making them swell, stick together and seal up as scar tissue. The injection produces a small localized sting or burning sensation that lasts a few seconds. The aim is to close off the affected vein and make the blood re-route through the normal veins – effectively improving the blood flow.

Following the injections, each injected site is covered with a pad and a stocking or bandage to hold it in place and apply compression. Such compression should be used for approximately 4 weeks, which makes it difficult to take a bath or shower. There are now special appliances (which look like a long plastic tube) that cover the bandage and seal up at the top, making showering possible. Alternatively, you could try using a bin bag secured at the top with a wide elastic band, wrapped around tightly enough to keep out the water, but not so tight as to hinder circulation. If the bandage does get damp, or if you find it uncomfortable, don't hesitate to ask for it to be reapplied by the nurse based at your local doctor's surgery.

By the time the bandage is removed, the treated vein should be far less prominent. However, the same vein may require more than one treatment. The improvement rate for injection sclerotherapy ranges from 50 to 90 per cent. Injection sclerotherapy is usually carried out at monthly intervals until the vein disappears. Most people require between two and four treatments.

The possible temporary side-effects include:

- stinging or cramping at the injection sites;
- raised red patches of skin at the injection sites;
- small skin sores or even a small ulcer at the injection sites;
- bruising at the injection sites;
- a rash at the injection sites;
- light ankle swelling (if you stand still for too long);
- groups of fine red blood vessels around the treated vein;
- brown lines around the treated vein.

To prevent the small risk of a blood clot developing in other leg veins – including the deep veins – the usual medical advice is to take a brisk walk or even a bike ride following injection sclerotherapy and to keep as active as possible thereafter. This reduces pressure and increases blood flow in the veins. It is also recommended that you avoid standing in one place for more than half an hour. When you need to be seated for a long period, it's a good idea to raise your legs. Of course, that may not be possible in your workplace, in which case – while you are seated – you should regularly lift your heels off the ground, then your toes (as described in Chapter 5). Moreover, it is important to take regular breaks to walk around.

While you are wearing the compression stockings or bandages in the weeks after treatment it is best to avoid strenuous activity that might loosen the bandages or cause injury. It is also advisable not to get into a squatting position to garden or do work of some kind, or to sit with your legs crossed or folded under you.

As well as the minimal risk of blood clots forming in additional leg veins, another possible but very rare complication of injection sclerotherapy and foam sclerotherapy (as explained below) is ulceration. Also, the chemicals used in sclerotherapy can cause an allergic reaction in the form of anaphylactic shock. Such a reaction is exceedingly rare but can be life-threatening. Fortunately, the medical team is normally prepared, ensuring that resuscitation equipment is to hand, just in case.

Foam sclerotherapy

If you suffer from larger varicose veins, the chemical used for injection sclerotherapy (see above) may be mixed with another chemical that froths to make a foam. Injections of foam spread faster through the veins and travel further. Foam sclerotherapy works in exactly the same way as injection sclerotherapy, the chemical causing the vein walls to collapse and stick together and the scar tissue then blocking off the vein. The injection is guided by ultrasound and is a relatively new technique. As with injection sclerotherapy, it carries the slight risk of blood clots in other veins. For that reason, after the procedure it's important to follow the exercise-related advice as given above.

There has been only one reported case of a stroke occurring after sclerotherapy treatment, when the patient concerned was given a very large dose of sclerosant foam

As with injection sclerotherapy, there is not yet sufficient available information to indicate how well this treatment works, how safe it is and which patients benefit most from it.

Endovenous laser therapy

Endovenous laser therapy (known as EVLT) is another means of closing an engorged superficial vein, causing the vein to shrink and its bulging appearance to disappear. The blood is diverted to normal veins and the flow becomes more efficient. After a local anaesthetic injection is administered, a laser fibre is inserted through a small needle hole in the skin into the affected vein. The laser is slowly heated, irritating the vein walls until the vein collapses. The procedure is carried out in a hospital out-patients department and takes up to 45 minutes.

There is always a very slight risk of deep vein thrombosis occurring after treatment to shut off a vein. However, the chances of this happening after EVLT are probably less than with any other procedure. To prevent DVT, you should wear compression stockings or bandages for a few weeks after treatment. The most common symptom after EVLT is numbness, which arises in a small number of cases. In a rare few, this can be a permanent feature. EVLT may cause minor soreness and bruising, but it leaves no visible scarring. Happily, there is generally immediate relief from varicose vein symptoms. Again, taking a brisk walk or bike ride after the procedure is your best course of action, with plenty of daily exercise thereafter.

Research has shown that, as well as minor soreness, other possible complications include the following:

- bruising: 24–100 per cent;
- burns: 4.8 per cent;
- tingling and numbness: 1–36.5 per cent;
- hardening along the saphenous vein: 55–100 per cent.

Radiofrequency occlusion

Radiofrequency occlusion (also known as the closure procedure) is an alternative treatment to the older and more traditional surgical stripping (see Chapter 9). The doctor uses an ultrasound machine to map the affected superficial vein. A small catheter is placed into the lower end of the vein through a small needle hole in the skin, after which radiofrequency waves are introduced. These waves cause the vein to heat up and collapse, making the vein gradually disappear, and with it the symptoms.

The procedure is performed on an out-patient basis, often under local anaesthetic. There is less post-operative pain, less bruising and a faster recovery period than with open surgery (see Chapter 9). The procedure takes about 45 minutes and again compression is provided in the form of stockings or bandages. Taking a brisk walk or bike ride afterwards is encouraged, as is regular activity thereafter. Squatting and 'pounding' exercise such as jogging are not recommended.

When a vascular expert looked closely at two controlled trials into radiofrequency occlusion compared with open surgery techniques, he found that after radiofrequency occlusion patients' recovery was speedier and there were fewer complications. Another vascular expert has written that open surgery for reflux in the small saphenous vein (SSV) is obsolete and that SSVs should be treated with non-invasive techniques, because of the high recurrence rates of the varicose veins after surgical intervention and the risk of nerve damage, possibly in up to 15 per cent of cases. In comparison, radio-frequency occlusion offers control in 80 per cent of cases of SSV reflux.

Like other varicose vein removal techniques, radiofrequency occlusion can cause complications, particularly if the advice to exercise is not followed. These include bruising, burns, tingling and phlebitis – all of which should clear up within a few weeks of treatment.

The figures for complications after this type of treatment sclerotherapy are fractionally higher than after open surgery:

- deep vein thrombosis: 0.57 per cent;
- pulmonary embolism: 0.17 per cent.

Hook phlebectomy

Hook phlebectomy (also known as ambulatory phlebectomy) is a means of physically taking away surface varicose veins in the leg that have not yet caused complications (as described in Chapter 3). Indeed, 'phlebectomy' means the physical removal of a vein. The procedure is minimally invasive and involves the surgeon making tiny incisions or needle punctures in the skin (as small as 1mm across) in order to extract the affected vein with an instrument known as a phlebectomy hook.

The procedure is usually carried out under local anaesthesia in the hospital out-patients department, but for some people a regional or general anaesthetic may be used. When local anaesthesia is used, the patient is able to walk immediately afterwards. The procedure is well tolerated by patients and produces good cosmetic results. Indeed, long-term results are excellent as long as the main source of the reflux is removed.

A compression bandage or stocking must be worn for a few weeks after treatment. As with other vascular treatments, you will be advised to take a brisk walk or bike ride when the procedure is over.

With hook phlebectomy there is less chance of the skin damage and discoloration that are linked with sclerotherapy. In contrast with traditional vein stripping, the small size of the incision or skin puncture results in little or no scarring. Moreover, because the procedure is usually carried out under local anaesthetic, the risks of a full anaesthetic are minimized greatly.

Hook phlebectomy is different from ligation and stripping (see Chapter 9), which is used to remove larger, more troublesome veins.

Transilluminated powered phlebectomy

Transilluminated powered phlebectomy (known as TIPP) is a relatively new minimally invasive procedure that physically removes the affected vein from the leg. Like hook phlebectomy, TIPP can be performed under local, regional or general anaesthesia. It takes about 30 minutes. An endoscope – a flexible tube with a light on the end – is inserted through a small incision under the skin, illuminating the vein clusters that require removal. Next, a suction device with guarded blades is inserted under the skin at another incision at the other end of the varicose vein. This device is skilfully manipulated to cut the vein into small pieces that can then be suctioned out of the body.

After the procedure, more anaesthetic is injected into the area to minimize bruising, pain and clotting. Finally, the incisions are closed with sutures or surgical tape. As with other vein removal techniques, the patient needs to wear compression stockings or bandages for a few weeks after the procedure and should take regular exercise. When general anaesthesia is used, most patients wake up without any pain and are allowed home after about an hour. Normal activity is encouraged immediately, with a return to work within 2–3 days.

The National Institute for Health and Clinical Excellence (NICE) compared studies of TIPP and hook phlebectomy and found there was similar or less pain at 6 weeks and greater cosmetic satisfaction with TIPP. Moreover, fewer incisions are generally required for TIPP. Comparative data also pointed to fewer complications with TIPP. The complications – although rare – associated with both phlebectomy procedures include bruising, tingling and numbness caused by nerve damage, as well as haematoma (a collection of blood under the skin). In one study of 114 patients, there was only one case of DVT – an aggregate of 0.9 per cent.

However, according to NICE, there is still insufficient good-quality evidence to be certain of how well TIPP works.

9

Vein ligation and stripping

Vein ligation and stripping involves tying the affected varicose vein so that blood can no longer flow through it – the word 'ligate' means to tie. Your vascular surgeon will advise you whether local anaesthetic or a general anaesthetic would be your best option. Whichever you choose, the procedure will be carried out in the operating room at your local hospital. Even if a general anaesthetic is used, you may be discharged on the day of surgery.

Prior to vein ligation and stripping, you will be asked to stand up for a while so the surgeon can see where the blood is pooling in your veins. The affected veins will be marked clearly with a pen because the bulges are not so evident when you are lying on the operating table. You are liable to be asked to shave your legs before the procedure, or a nurse may do it for you.

Ligation and stripping are generally carried out on larger, more troublesome varicose veins, when vein complications have occurred, or when your surgeon considers complications to be a threat. These complications are discussed in Chapter 3 and include ankle swelling, vein rupture, thrombophlebitis (sometimes just referred to as phlebitis), venous eczema, skin damage (including discoloration) and ulceration. According to one study of venous ulcers, 28 per cent of people who used only compression treatment suffered at least one further ulcer compared with 14 per cent who underwent vein ligation and stripping in combination with compression treatment.[1]

After the procedure, your surgeon may recommend that you have sclerotherapy on any smaller incompetent veins. In a massive 90 per cent of patients, vein ligation and stripping produces good-to-excellent long-term results. Each year in England and Wales, about 50,000 people have varicose vein surgery.

The benefits of ligation and stripping

To date, little reliable research into the benefits of varicose vein surgery has been carried out. The data that we do have, however, show the following:

- there is an improvement in symptoms such as aching and heaviness;[2]
- your legs have a better appearance;[3]
- you will enjoy life more.[4]

In one study carried out in patients a few months after varicose vein surgery, nearly 90 per cent of respondents said that their legs were 'much better' or 'cured'. After 10 years, two thirds of these people said their legs still looked and felt better.[5] In another study carried out in patients 6 months after surgery, 80 per cent stated that their quality of life had improved, that they felt less self-conscious, that they could wear clothes that showed their legs and that they could perform daily tasks and play sport more comfortably.[6]

I should point out, though, that not everyone is happy with the results of surgery. Two out of 10 of the post-varicose vein surgery population is still a high amount – and this number were disappointed with how their legs looked and felt. Similarly, one out of 10 complained that there was not a significant reduction in their symptoms, such as aching and heaviness. However, experts such as consultant vascular surgeon Professor Bruce Campbell of the Royal Devon and Exeter Hospital feel that, properly performed, surgery has good long-term results with low levels of complications.

At the hospital

Local anaesthetic

If you have a heart condition, a tendency to developing blood clots or some other health problem, a general anaesthetic, which makes you sleep during surgery, may not be recommended. Under local anaesthetic, you remain awake throughout the procedure and receive injections of an anaesthetic medication in your legs to make them numb. You will not feel pain during surgery and you'll be aware of what's going on around you. A nurse or anaesthetist will talk to you throughout the procedure to help to keep you calm.

General anaesthetic

General anaesthesia is a state of total unconsciousness resulting from a variety of anaesthetic drugs that are given to the patient. These drugs have different effects with the overall aim of ensuring that:

- the patient remains unconsciousness throughout the procedure;
- the patient has no memory of the procedure;
- no pain is felt during the procedure.

Anaesthetists are skilled at selecting the optimum technique for any given patient and procedure. If you are being given a general anaesthetic, you will not be able to eat or drink for 6–8 hours before the operation. It is important that you have an empty stomach when you are under a general anaesthetic because it makes you less likely to vomit, and vomiting while unconscious is dangerous because the reflex to cough is lost; as a result, some of the stomach contents can get into the lungs. Some anaesthetists allow their patients to take a few sips of water until 2 hours before the operation.

Preparing for the operation

In some cases, you may be asked to meet your anaesthetist in a pre-admission clinic a few days before the operation. However, most people don't meet their anaesthetist until the day of the surgery. The anaesthetist will ask:

- about your general health;
- whether you have allergies or suffer from hay fever, asthma or eczema;
- what any previous experience of anaesthesia was like;
- what medications you are taking (whether prescribed or over-the-counter);
- whether you smoke.

If you smoke, you would be best advised to give up a few weeks before surgery. This will minimize your risk of breathing problems during and after general anaesthesia.

If you have dental crowns, bridges or loose teeth, you should tell your anaesthetist. He or she will then try to protect them from being damaged by the tube that is put in your mouth while you are unconscious.

On the day of your admission, you should remove any nail polish, make-up and jewellery. If you prefer not to take off your rings, a nurse will cover them with sticky tape. You will also need to remove such things as contact lenses, glasses, dentures and hearing aids. They will be kept safe for you until you come round from the operation.

It is normal to feel nervous before any surgical procedure. The anaesthetist will ask how anxious you feel and may offer a pre-medication drug to calm your nerves. If you are not asked and you are feeling anxious, don't hesitate to speak up.

In the operating theatre

You will be wheeled to the operating theatre on a gurney or stretcher bed where an assistant will help to prepare you for surgery. A narrow plastic tube called a cannula will be inserted into a vein, usually on the back of your hand or in your arm. This feels rather like an injection and soon settles down. The anaesthetist now administers the various drugs, through the cannula, that render you unconscious and control pain and nausea. Within seconds you will fall asleep, after which a drip to keep you hydrated may be set up, with the fluid entering your body through the cannula. You will remain asleep throughout the procedure, and the anaesthetist will stay with you, keeping a careful watch on the machines that monitor the activity of your heart and other body systems. He or she will also constantly watch your heart rate, blood pressure and the amount of oxygen in your bloodstream.

Waking up

After the anaesthetic is stopped, you will begin to wake up and the tube will be removed from your throat. You will be moved to the recovery room and given one-to-one care by a nurse who is likely to administer oxygen through a face-mask and who will monitor your heart rate, blood pressure and other vital functions.

It is normal to feel sleepy or disorientated for 15 minutes or so after starting to wake.

Ligation and stripping – the procedure

When you are unconscious, the vascular surgeon will begin to work on the veins that have been found to be incompetent and that were earlier marked out on your leg in pen.

The long saphenous vein (LSV)

If the LSV was deemed to be incompetent, the surgeon will make an incision in the skin crease of the groin – in a very slim patient it may be only 2cm in length and in a very overweight patient it may be 5cm in length.

The LSV is positioned in the fatty layer beneath the skin. To stop blood flowing through the vein, the small branches leading off from it are all located and tied off – the process called ligation. Next, the LSV is freed down to its junction with the main deep vein and is also tied off. The surgeon leaves a surgical clip here on the lower end of the vein. Next, a thin flexible wire or fine metal rod known as a 'vein stripper' is threaded down the inside of the vein. As the vein comes out, it is turned inside out – a process called inversion stripping.

Sometimes, a second, smaller incision is made lower down the leg, usually on the inside of the knee. However, if you are having the entire vein removed, the second incision will be made at the ankle. A stripping tool at the end of the flexible wire pulls the vein through the second incision. The surgeon now sews up the wound (or wounds) using stitches that slowly dissolve as the wound heals.

When the main LSV has been taken away, incisions are made at the sites of other smaller varicose veins that were marked before the procedure, as discussed in the Chapter 8 in the section on 'hook phlebectomy' (see page 78). Those veins are then stripped, too, using the hook implement. To reduce bleeding as the veins are removed – smaller ones may not bleed, but very large ones can bleed a lot – the ends of the veins are likely to be tied by the surgeon or sealed using sticky paper strips. Another option is for the surgeon to apply a special tourniquet to the thigh to prevent bleeding. Yet another option is for the surgeon to wrap a bandage around the leg from the foot upwards in order to halt blood loss.

When the procedure is over, the whole leg is bandaged.

The short saphenous vein (SSV)

Using duplex scanning or hand-held Doppler ultrasound (see Chapter 7) the surgeon will mark the upper end of an incompetent SSV prior to ligation and stripping. A varicose SSV needs to be tied off at its junction with the main deep vein, which lies just above the back of the knee. The patient will lie on his or her stomach for the duration of the operation, but this makes general anaesthesia a little more difficult because the anaesthetic cannot be delivered through a face mask, but must be provided through a special device called an endotracheal tube or a laryngeal mask.

The surgeon's next step is to make a 3–4cm incision behind the knee in order to locate the SSV. The vein is dissected down to its junction with the main deep vein before being tied off and divided. In comparison with the LSV, the SSV is not routinely stripped. However, stripping may be used if the vein is very bulky. In most cases, phlebectomy (see page 78) is carried out to remove the vein.

If the LSV also requires surgery, the patient will be turned over at this point.

The perforator veins

When investigation has shown the perforator veins to be incompetent, they need to be tied off and phlebectomies carried out. Perforators in the calf are now usually dealt with by a procedure known as subfascial endoscopic perforator surgery, in which a flexible telescope is passed through small incisions to enable the surgeon to view the tissue beneath the skin. To improve access, a space-maker balloon is fed through the telescope and then inflated. The varicose perforator veins are tied off with endoscopic scissors, or sealed with an ultrasonic coagulator called an harmonic scalpel.

Only a small number of people have perforator veins that need surgical treatment. The procedure is generally carried out after the saphenous veins have been treated, as described above.

When the procedure is finished, the leg will be bandaged.

Are the leg veins needed in the case of heart by-pass?

Because the LSV is often used as a replacement or graft for an artery in the heart during heart by-pass surgery, there was once concern about removing it. The truth is, though, that an incompetent varicose vein would not work as a vein graft anyway so medical professionals believe there is no reason not to strip it.

When the LSV is absent or damaged, a blood vessel from the chest – called the mammary artery – can be used during heart by-pass surgery. In some cases, even the arm veins have been used with great success.

After ligation and stripping

When the procedure is over and you have woken up after the effects of the general anaesthetic have worn off, you are likely to have a cannula in the back of your hand or in your arm where you were given the anaesthetic. As soon as you feel up to it, you should ask a nurse if you can try to have a walk around the ward. This gets the blood pumping through your leg veins and helps to protect against blood clots (thrombosis).

Some people are slow to be up and about if they have had extensive surgery on both legs or if they have other medical problems. The advice for such people is to take several short walks – maybe just walking around the bed or across to the next bed and back – rather than trying to walk the length of the ward in one go. Try your best to be as active as possible, and you will feel the benefit. When you aren't walking you should try to elevate your feet, placing them higher than your hips.

Before your discharge from hospital, you will probably receive written advice about what to do if you encounter problems. You will also be given a letter to hand to your general practitioner. If a stocking needs to be substituted for bandages the next day, arrangements for this will be made in advance.

Slim patients who have only had one leg operated on and little bruising may feel they are back to normal within 3 weeks, whereas overweight patients with surgery to both legs may feel it takes 2–3 months to recover fully. The ankles may remain swollen for a long time after the bruising has settled, and the scarring can take many months to fade. In a few cases, a brownish stain appears in the area where the vein was removed. Another rare complication is the appearance of tiny blue veins on neighbouring areas of skin.

Pain and discomfort

Most people would say they felt discomfort rather than pain after the surgery. However, owing mainly to chemical and genetic factors, we all have different pain levels and for a small number of people the post-operative pain is the worst they have experienced. If the painkillers you are given don't seem to be working, tell your nurse, who will be able to give you a higher dosage or a different painkiller.

Obviously, it will be easier to walk if you have only had one leg operated on rather than both. The general consensus is that the incision at the groin is the cause of most discomfort because it is a deeper wound than the others. In very overweight people, the wound is deeper still and is therefore more uncomfortable than in a very slim person. Surgeons sometimes use additional local anaesthetic at the groin, which can result in far less discomfort than would otherwise be experienced.

In the following few days, as more bruising comes out, there can be a greater awareness of aches and pains. Where the LSV was stripped, in the lower part of the inner thigh, there can be increasing tenderness and stiffness after activity. It is important not to let this stop you being active. In the early days, it is preferable to take painkillers and continue to build up your activity levels slowly rather than being inactive and not take painkillers – however much you may dislike taking tablets. You will be provided with painkillers while you are still in hospital, and you are likely to be sent home with a prescription for more. Painkillers such as ibuprofen and paracetamol can also be purchased at chemists and even supermarkets.

The wounds

During the first 24 hours after surgery, the incisions that were made and closed with adhesive strips may ooze a little blood. This oozing usually stops on its own, but if it doesn't and you are now at home you can gently press on the wound for a few minutes with a clean dressing, a cotton wool ball or a large folded tissue. In most cases, the bleeding will stop. If it doesn't, you should ring your hospital ward for advice. You may be asked to go to the hospital to have the wound cleaned and re-closed.

To prevent the wound at the groin becoming sweaty and unpleasant, you will be able to wash it after a couple of days. Any wounds that were so tiny they did not require closing with adhesive strips or dressing in any way should be kept dry for 7–10 days. Obviously, bathing is very difficult when you are not able to get your legs wet, but people who have only had one leg operated on can get round this problem by sitting in shallow water and propping their leg on the side of the bath. If both legs have undergone surgery, you can take a shower by stepping into a couple of large bin liners and securing the tops with wide rubber bands. There are also surgical appliance manufacturers who sell plastic leg bags and special fastenings that keep out the water when you are taking a shower.

Bandages and support stockings

You are likely to wake up from surgery wearing bandages around your legs (or around one leg if only one leg was operated on). The bandages are usually changed for special support stockings the next day. If you find them reasonably comfortable, you should wear them all the time – otherwise you can remove them at night just before getting into bed and put them on again the next morning as soon as you get out of bed.

It is required that you wear support stockings for about 10 days after surgery. However, your surgeon is likely to recommend that you wear them for longer if they make your legs feel more comfortable.

Lumpiness and bruising

Lumpiness and bruising arise as a result of blood running into the areas where the veins were removed. Larger veins create larger spaces and are therefore associated with more lumpiness and bruising. The lumps are actually collections of blood that have formed into clots, whereas the bruising comes from blood spreading out in the spaces beneath the skin. The blood clots harden with time and present no risk, and the bruising disappears slowly over a month or more. The inner part of the thigh is usually the site of most lumpiness and bruising. It can feel very tender for a few days after the operation. The lumps are usually absorbed by the body over a period of several weeks.

You will wake up from the surgery wearing bandages or compression stockings which, if they continue to be worn, reduce the amount of lumpiness and bruising. If your surgeon prescribes warfarin or heparin to minimize the small risk of deep vein thrombosis, the blood is less liable to clot, but there is generally more bruising.

Patches of tiny red veins

In the days and weeks after surgery, clumps of tiny red veins known as 'matting' can appear on the skin in the areas that were operated on. Six out of 10 people had this problem in one study of the after-effects of hook phlebectomy.[7]

The importance of being active

If surgery has been performed on the groin area, getting up from a seat may cause discomfort for a few days. The leg may feel tender in places, and there is likely to be stiffness on walking. However, walking is the best medicine and you should try to move around every half hour during the day for the first couple of weeks after surgery. In the past, doctors used to tell their post-operative varicose vein patients to walk 3 miles a day, but walking a long distance is no longer recommended. It is more important to take frequent short walks than struggling to take longer ones, especially in the early days. When your legs are feeling more comfortable, you can take longer walks, if you wish.

If you are keen to get back to a taxing activity such as field and racket sports, don't do so until you no longer need to wear bandages or support stockings. You can then gradually ease yourself back into your old way of life – perhaps the things you used to do before your vein problems slowed you down. Don't return to swimming, however, until the wounds on your legs are dry and healed.

It is recommended that, if you drive a car, you wait for a week to 10 days before getting behind the wheel once more. Ask your doctor's advice, however, on when you can go back to work – you may need a couple of weeks or so off. It is all right to have sex as soon as you feel able to.

Possible complications of surgery

Risks are attached to all operations; these risks include infection, bleeding and the risks from anaesthesia (see page 92). With vein ligation and stripping, there is a possibility of the veins recurring, infection of the wound, lymphatic discharge, nerve damage, fluid build-up, swelling, bleeding and scarring. In one study of 600 people, one in six had a problem after varicose vein surgery. These included such things as swelling, bruising and blisters caused by the bandages rubbing their skin.[8]

Complications related to the wound at the groin are more likely in overweight people. Previous surgery in the groin area also raises the chances of complications occurring.

Surgery is carried out on a very limited basis in patients with problems in the deep veins as well as varicose veins because there is a greater risk of blood clots developing, as well as deep venous thrombosis.

Wound infection

Bacterial infection in one or more of the wounds can happen in some cases, particularly in the wound at the groin. This causes the area around the wound to hurt and the skin to be hot and red. When this wound has been closed by a stitch (suture) under the skin, the stitch may need to be removed to allow the infection to resolve itself. In a small number of cases, a groin abscess may develop and need to be opened up in an operation. A groin abscess will then need regular dressing until it heals.

One study found that an infection arose in less than one in 100 people.[9] Another found that 4 in 100 people were troubled by infection.[10]

Lymphatic discharge

A type of fluid known as lymph, which contains white blood cells, is carried around the tissues in tiny channels to the lymph glands in the groin. When a surgical procedure interferes with these lymph glands at the groin, they generally seal off automatically. However, sometimes one will not seal off but instead begins producing a discharge of lymph or a collection of clear fluid that forms into a lump. The discharge or lump will usually clear up without treatment.

Nerve damage

It is fairly common for nerves beneath the skin to be damaged during surgery to remove varicose veins. The result is one or more patches of numbness on the leg and ankle. These numb patches usually shrink or completely disappear over time. There is a far greater risk of nerve damage occurring when varicose veins on the foot are stripped, and this, in turn, causes a larger patch of numbness. Surgery to remove varicose veins behind the knee can, in a tiny percentage of people, damage the main nerves that move the leg and foot.

If a nerve has merely been bruised or stretched, it will recover over time. If it has been cut, however, it will never completely recover. Fortunately, few people find permanent numbness a problem.

Leg or ankle swelling

Varicose vein surgery can result in swelling of the leg, in particular in the ankle area. The likelihood of this happening is greater if you have undergone previous varicose vein surgery or if your legs or ankles have a tendency to swell anyway. Post-operative swelling is caused by disturbance to the lymphatic tubes that lie close to the varicose veins and drain lymph (see the previous page) upwards from the foot and leg.

In most cases, the swelling takes several weeks to settle and for some the swelling remains a permanent feature.

Fluid build-up

In some cases, a build-up of fluid can occur near the groin wound. The fluid can leak out of it, making it feel wet and uncomfortable. Your surgeon might advise having the fluid drained off.

Bleeding

After surgery, the incisions that were made in your skin can bleed. If the bleeding is fairly substantial, blood clots will form and the area will swell and feel tender. The result is a large bruise called a haematoma, which may require further surgery.

Deep vein thrombosis

When deep vein thrombosis (DVT) occurs, the affected leg swells and a blood clot can work its way up to the lungs – a situation that results in pulmonary embolism. In people who are at higher risk of DVT – women who take the contraceptive pill, for example – injections of a drug called heparin may be administered. Heparin is a blood-thinning agent that helps to stop the blood clotting; however, it therefore creates more bruising than would otherwise occur.

The risk of DVT can be reduced significantly by moving around after the surgery, and thereafter taking regular short walks. Women who take the contraceptive pill are likely to be given the pros and cons of coming off it temporarily before the surgery.

Damage to major arteries or deep veins

Damage to the major arteries or the deep veins has occurred in the past during varicose vein surgery. This damage can result in severe loss of blood and even death. Fortunately, surgeons are very aware of this miniscule risk and take every precaution to ensure that it doesn't happen.

Foot drop

In a tiny number of cases, the big nerve that runs down the back of the thigh is damaged in surgery. This makes the foot weak and floppy – a condition called 'foot drop'.

The risks from general anaesthesia

General anaesthesia is usually very safe these days. Its most common complications are problems that quickly pass, such as nausea, vomiting, a sore throat and hoarseness. However, the vast majority of patients experience no after-effects, barring a little sleepiness that soon wears off.

More serious complications, such as brain damage and death are extremely rare, but slightly more likely in people who have a heart condition or who have had a previous blood clot. Complications occur so infrequently that the chances of them happening have been difficult to measure with certainty. Moreover, surgeons and anaesthetists take every precaution to keep the risk of serious complications as low as possible. If the patient is otherwise healthy and not greatly overweight, varicose vein surgery is classed as low risk. If your overall health is not good, or if you have a heart condition or a tendency to blood clotting, you are likely to have a local anaesthetic and so be awake but with your legs numbed for the surgery (see page 81).

Can the varicose veins reappear?

Whether a person develops new varicose veins in the years after surgery depends largely on the thoroughness of the operation and the diagnostic procedure before it. In one study of people who had undergone surgery for varicose veins, the veins had reappeared in 3 out of 10 people after 5 years, and in 4 out of 10 people after 10 years.[11] The use of duplex ultrasound investigation has lowered the incidence of recurrence, but the technique is so new that as yet no studies into its long-term effectiveness have been completed.

Veins that have been tied off are more likely to return than veins that have been removed in some way. If only a part of the vein has been removed – from the knee downwards, for instance – there is also more likelihood of the varicosity returning. Surgeons are not always willing to remove the whole vein, however, because it carries a higher risk of nerve damage. One study indicated that there is less chance of veins coming back if the surgeon uses a combination of vein stripping and removing the perforator veins through small incisions.[12]

10

Complementary therapies

Many people with varicose veins try complementary therapies. However, some types of therapy can cause adverse reactions, and the quality and strength of complementary therapies is not controlled by a regulating body. In comparison with mainstream medicine, in which there has been a great deal of research, there has been little research and few controlled scientific trials into the effects of complementary medicine. Before you decide to try a particular therapy, it is recommended that you find out as much as you can about it. You could also ask your doctor's advice.

Complementary remedies are unlikely to make varicose veins go away completely. That said, some people with varicose veins who use complementary therapies report great benefits. The benefits may, to some extent, come from people knowing that they are doing something positive to help themselves. However, there is no doubt that the more relaxing complementary therapies can reduce the stress that can be caused by cosmetic concerns or by the symptoms and complications of varicose veins.

Acupuncture

An ancient form of oriental healing, acupuncture involves puncturing the skin with fine needles at specific points in the body. These points are located along energy channels (meridians) that are believed to correspond with certain internal organs. This energy is known as chi. Needles are inserted to increase, decrease or unblock the flow of chi energy so that the balance of yin and yang is restored.

Yin, the female force, is calm and passive; it also represents dark, cold, swelling and moisture. On the other hand, yang, the male force, is stimulating and aggressive, representing heat, light, contraction and dryness. It is thought that an imbalance in these forces is the cause of illness and disease. For example, a person who feels the cold, suffers fluid retention and fatigue would be considered to have an excess of yin. A person suffering from repeated headaches, however, will be deemed to have an excess of yang. Emotional, physical or environmental factors are believed to disturb the chi energy balance, and can also be treated.

A qualified acupuncturist will use a set method to determine acupuncture points – it is thought there are as many as 2,000 acupuncture points on the body. At a consultation, questions may be asked about lifestyle, sleeping patterns, fears, phobias and reactions to stress. The pulses will be felt, after which the acupuncture itself is carried out, fine needles being placed at the relevant sites. The first consultation will normally last for an hour, and the client should notice a change for the better after four to six sessions.

Acupuncturists claim to be able to improve varicose veins by boosting the circulation. By treating key points along the meridians, blood is said to be forced to move through the veins and surrounding areas. Points that may boost energy and blood flow are usually worked on, too. Acupuncturists liken treatment for varicosities to a clogged pipe being washed wide open by a forceful gush of water.

The person being treated will normally experience tingling or a heavy distended sensation. Some people have reported an itching sensation as the blood in the veins is believed to start moving. Acupuncturists say that improvements are seen gradually, with varicosities becoming lighter in colour and spreading out over a wider area before disappearing. It is believed that the more treatment a person receives, the more progress will be made. However, the healing process can also be hastened by hydrotherapy (see pages 105–6), the daily application of apple cider vinegar (see page 103) and the use of herbal remedies, as well as by self-help measures (see Chapter 5).

Acupuncture is a safe therapy. The only very slight risk is that of infection from the needles.

Aromatherapy

Apparently, certain health disorders can be treated by stimulating our sense of smell with aromatic oils – known as essential oils. Once the sense of smell has been stimulated, it is believed that a particular smell can help to treat a particular health problem. There's no doubt at all that aromatherapy can aid relaxation and help to reduce anxiety, tension and depression, all of which can arise in a person with varicose veins.

Concentrated essential oils are extracted from plants and may be inhaled, rubbed directly into the skin or used in bathing. Each odour relates to its plant of origin – so, for example, lavender oil has the aroma of the lavender plant, and geranium has the aroma of the geranium plant.

Plant essences have been used for healing throughout the ages, smaller amounts being used for aromatherapy purposes than for herbal medicines. The highly concentrated aromatherapy oils are obtained either by steaming a particular plant extract until the oil glands burst, or by soaking the plant extract in hot oil so that the cells collapse and release their essence.

Techniques used in aromatherapy

There are several ways of using aromatherapy, the main ones being:

- Inhalation, which gives the fastest result. The inhalation of essential oils has a direct influence on the olfactory (nasal) organs, and signals are immediately received by the brain. Steam inhalation is the most popular technique. This can be achieved either by mixing a few drops of oil with a bowlful of boiling water, or by using an oil burner whereby the flame from a tea-light candle heats a small saucer of water containing a few drops of oil.
- Massage, which normally uses essential oils that have been pre-diluted (oils intended for massage should never be applied to the skin in an undiluted or pure form). When using undiluted essential oils, mix three or four drops with a neutral carrier oil such as olive or safflower oil. After they have penetrated the skin, the oils are absorbed by the body. The oils are believed to exert a positive influence on a particular organ or set of tissues.
- Bathing. Tension and anxiety can be reduced by using aromatherapy oils in the bath. A few drops of pure essential oil should

be added directly to running tap water – the oil mixes with the water more efficiently this way. No more than 20 drops of oil in total should be used.

Oils for relaxation

Lavender is the most popular oil for relaxation. It is known to be a wonderful restorative and it is excellent for relieving tension headaches as well as stress. However, there are several others that, when used alone or blended, can provide a relaxing atmosphere – Roman chamomile and ylang ylang, for example. Ylang ylang has relaxing properties and a calming effect on the heart rate, and it can relieve palpitations and raised blood pressure. Chamomile can be very soothing, too, and aids both sleep and digestion.

Drop relaxation oils into the vessel part of the burner and top up with water. Light the tea-light candle and try to relax while the essential oils scent the whole room – don't let the water evaporate totally. Such oils are safe around babies and children, because rather than being overpowering, the aroma is soft and soothing.

Various recipes for relaxation oils exist:

Recipe 1
- 5 drops of lavender,
- 2 drops of Roman chamomile,
- 1 drop of ylang ylang.

Blend well and diffuse in a burner.

Recipe 2
- 8 drops of mandarin,
- 3 drops of neroli,
- 3 drops of ylang ylang.

Blend well and diffuse in a burner.

Recipe 3
- 10 drops of bergamot,
- 2 drops of rose otto,
- 3 drops of Roman chamomile.

Blend well and diffuse in a burner.

Recipe 4

For relaxation, this is a great blend for use in the bath.

- 3 drops of lavender,
- 2 drops of marjoram,
- 2 drops of basil,
- 1 drop of vetiver,
- 1 drop of fennel.

Recipes 2 and 3 can also be added to 50ml (2 fluid ounces) of distilled water, shaken well and used in a spray bottle for a room freshener with relaxing properties.

For a person with varicose veins, the essential oils palmarosa, myrtle, chamomile, cypress, juniper berry, myrrh and frankincense can be of benefit, reducing enlarged veins, easing inflammation and lessening pain. Massage oils containing any of these ingredients can be rubbed on the veins – but be careful not to rub too hard on veins that are already fragile. In massaging the legs, always stroke upwards towards the heart.

If the skin has broken and a varicose ulcer has formed, it is recommended that you apply a compress of lavender essential oil to the area. Where the varicose veins are swollen and inflamed, carrot seed essential oil – used as a compress – can be of great benefit. This oil can be difficult to find, however, and may need to be ordered.

Other recipes:

- 3 drops of chamomile oil, 3 drops of carrot seed oil, 3 drops of lavender oil, 1 cup of cold water, 1 teaspoon of tincture of calendula or St John's wort. After mixing the ingredients together, stir in a soft cloth, wring it out and place it over the itching or broken varicose veins as often as you can – preferably on a daily basis. The tinctures can be purchased from health food shops.
- 10 drops of palmarosa oil, 8 drops of cypress oil, 7 drops of chamomile oil, 25g (1 fluid ounce) of vegetable oil or St John's wort. After mixing the ingredients together, stir in a soft cloth, wring it out and place it over the problem veins as often as you can – preferably on a daily basis. This recipe works best when added to infused oil of St John's wort, which can be purchased from health food shops.

Seeing an aromatherapist

Because aromatherapy is a holistic therapy (where the practitioner looks at the person and his or her ills as a whole), the therapist will ask questions on lifestyle, family circumstances and so on. Depending upon your answers, a suitable blend of oils will be recommended and a back massage offered. As well as often being beneficial health-wise, aromatherapy massages are very relaxing. If you are unable to consult with a qualified aromatherapist, your local health food shop may provide you with details of which essential oils are appropriate for your needs. Alternatively, you may want to borrow a good aromatherapy book from your nearest library.

Biofeedback

In biofeedback, people are taught how to listen to what their bodies are telling them for the good of their health. For instance, an anxious person is taught how to recognize muscle tension, irritability and palpitations as the onset of an anxiety attack. After being shown how to relax by the biofeedback tecnhique, the person should see real benefits in their health.

In the late 1960s, when the term 'biofeedback' was first coined, research showed that certain involuntary actions like heart rate, blood pressure and brain function can be altered by tuning into the body. For instance, many people calm their anxiety by reading an interesting book. As a result, their heart stops racing and their blood pressure falls to more normal levels. Later research has shown that biofeedback can help in the treatment of many diseases and painful conditions, and that we have more control over so-called involuntary function than we once thought possible. Scientists are now trying to determine just how much voluntary control we can exert.

Biofeedback is now widely used to treat pain, high and low blood pressure, paralysis, epilepsy and many other disorders. The technique is taught by psychiatrists, psychologists, doctors and physiotherapists.

A biofeedback specialist will normally teach people with a pain problem the following techniques:

- a relaxation technique;
- how to identify the circumstances that trigger (or worsen) their symptoms;
- how to cope with events they have previously avoided due to their symptoms;
- how to set attainable goals;
- how to regain control of their life.

Users of biofeedback must learn to examine their day-to-day lives in order to ascertain whether they are somehow contributing to their health problem. They must recognize that they can, by their own efforts, get far more out of their lives. In the correct use of biofeedback, bad habits must be changed and, most importantly, the user must accept much of the responsibility for maintaining his or her own health.

Scientists believe that relaxation is the key to the success of this technique. The person is taught to react with a calmer frame of mind to certain stimuli – the appearance of the varicose veins when they look in a mirror, for instance. As a result, the stress response is not triggered and adrenalin is not pumped into the bloodstream. Without biofeedback training, adrenalin may be released repeatedly causing chronic anxiety, stress, muscle tension and depression.

If you think you might benefit from biofeedback training, you should discuss the matter with your doctor or other health care professional.

Herbal remedies

There are several herbal remedies that are known to be effective in the treatment of varicose veins.

Horse chestnut (*Aesculus hippocastanum*)

A series of studies have shown that taking horse chestnut capsules can help to increase blood flow up and out of the legs, strengthen connective tissues and vein walls, reduce redness and swelling and relieve painful leg conditions caused by poor circulation. The active ingredient in horse chestnut is a compound known as *Aescin*. Aescin appears to block the release of enzymes that damage capillary walls. Horse chestnut is therefore an excellent treatment for varicose veins. Take horse chestnut capsules containing 50–300mg of Aescin two or three times a day or 1–5 drops of horse chestnut tincture three times a day. It may take up to 6 weeks to see improvements.

This herb should be avoided by people with kidney or liver disease and during pregnancy and breast-feeding.

Witch hazel

Extracted from the leaves and bark of the witch hazel plant, witch hazel is used externally to ease bruising, sores and swelling. Apply twice a day to the affected veins, or take 10–60 drops of witch hazel tincture four times a day. Witch hazel ointment and tinctures are available from health food shops. Results may not be seen for 2–3 weeks. The ointment may cause minor irritation in some people.

Pycnogenol

Made from pine bark extract, pycnogenol has anti-inflammatory properties and can be of significant benefit to circulatory disorders. Take 100mg three times daily for 2 months then reduce the dosage.

Butcher's broom

Butcher's broom is a member of the lily family. It contains ruscogenins – constituents that are believed to strengthen the collagen in blood vessel walls and boost circulation. Weak, dilated blood vessels – such as varicose veins – can therefore be tightened and so cause fewer symptoms. The side-effects of butcher's broom can include indigestion and nausea.

You should consult your doctor before taking this herb as it may have a negative effect on certain conditions, including high blood pressure, and it should be avoided in pregnancy and breast-feeding. Butcher's broom is available from health food shops.

Grape seed and pine bark extracts

The extract of grape seeds and pine bark contain compounds that appear to strengthen the connective tissue structure of blood vessels and reduce inflammation. It is therefore recommended for people with varicose veins. The side-effects can include indigestion and nausea.

Because of its effects on the immune system, people with autoimmune conditions, such as rheumatoid arthritis, multiple sclerosis and Crohn's disease, should only take pine bark or grape seed extract under a doctor's supervision. Medications that suppress the immune system should not be taken with pine bark or grape seed extract, and these extracts should not be combined with corticosteroids, unless under medical supervision. The safety of these extracts has not been established in children and pregnant or breast-feeding women.

Gotu kola

The herb gotu kola appears to be effective at strengthening connective tissue (including vein walls) and boosting circulation. Indeed, several studies have indicated that gotu kola extract can significantly improve varicose vein symptoms, reducing swelling, pain, the sensation of heaviness and fluid leakage from the veins. However, as yet, no studies have ascertained whether gotu kola can actually make visible varicose veins disappear, or prevent new ones from developing.

It is recommended that you consult your doctor before taking this herb. Its safety for pregnant and breast-feeding women, children and people with liver or kidney disease has not been established.

Gotu kola is available from health food shops. Follow the label dosage instructions and allow at least 4 weeks for the herb to begin working.

Ginkgo biloba

This herb is capable of improving the circulation and strengthening blood vessels. It may therefore be of benefit to people with varicose veins.

Ginkgo biloba can be purchased in capsule form from health food shops, some pharmacies and the larger supermarkets, and the label dosage instructions should be followed. This herb is usually well tolerated, but consult your doctor beforehand if you are taking prescribed medication – particularly warfarin, heparin or aspirin – because dangerous bleeding can occur.

Hawthorn

Hawthorn is excellent for boosting the circulatory system, strengthening blood vessels and reducing swelling and inflammation. It is a safe and gentle herb to take and can be used over a long period of time. This herb is available from health food shops and the label dosage instructions should be followed.

It is possible to make a tea (or herbal infusion) from natural hawthorn, to be drunk three times a day. Pour a cup of water over 2 teaspoons of crushed berries or flowers and leaves, cover and steep for 20 minutes. Strain and drink.

Apple cider vinegar

People with varicose veins have reported significant benefits from using apple cider vinegar. There are two ways to use this product:

- using a cupped hand, apply undiluted apple cider vinegar to the area over the varicose veins and massage well in – stroking towards the heart from the ankle upward to the knee and then the thigh – and repeat every morning and night;
- take apple cider vinegar with honey three times a day – mix 2 teaspoons of cider vinegar with 2 teaspoons of honey in a glassful of water and drink.

After 4–6 weeks, you should notice that your veins are beginning to shrink.

Aloe vera gel

Aloe vera is a plant with thick, fleshy leaves that has long been used externally to treat skin conditions such as cuts, burns and eczema. It is believed also to ease pain and reduce inflammation. Therefore, itchy and irritated varicose veins can be soothed by applying aloe vera gel. Pain and swelling can also be eased. Aloe vera is often mixed with other useful compounds and is widely available.

Topical applications

Applying chamomile, comfrey, oatstraw or white oak bark – in ointment form – to varicose veins can significantly reduce symptoms.

Homoeopathy

The homoeopathic approach to medicine is holistic – that is, the overall health of a person, physical, emotional and psychological, is assessed before treatment is started. The homoeopathic belief is that the whole make-up of a person determines the disorders to which he or she is prone and the symptoms that are likely to occur. After a thorough consultation, the homoeopath will offer a remedy compatible with the patient's symptoms as well as with the patient's temperament and characteristics. Consequently, two people with the same disorder may be offered entirely different remedies.

Homoeopathic remedies are derived from plant, mineral and animal substances, which are soaked in alcohol to extract the 'live' ingredients. This initial solution is then diluted many times and shaken vigorously after each dilution to add energy. Impurities are removed and the remaining solution is made up into tablets, ointments, powders or suppositories. Low-dilution remedies are used for severe symptoms whereas high-dilution remedies are used for milder symptoms.

The homoeopathic concept has, since antiquity, been that 'like cures like'. The full healing abilities of this type of remedy were first recognized in the early nineteenth century when the German doctor Samuel Hahnemann noticed that the herbal cure for malaria – which was based on an extract of cinchona bark (quinine) – actually produced symptoms of malaria. Further tests convinced him that the production of mild symptoms caused the body to fight the disease. He went on to treat malaria patients successfully with dilute doses of cinchona bark.

Each homoeopathic remedy is first 'proved' by being taken by a healthy person – usually a volunteer homoeopath – and the symptoms noted. This remedy is said to be capable of curing the same symptoms in an ill person. The whole idea of 'proving' and using homoeopathic remedies can be difficult to comprehend, because it is exactly the opposite of how conventional medicines operate. For example, a patient who has a cold with a runny nose would be treated with a homoeopathic remedy that would produce a runny nose in a healthy patient. Conventional medicine, on the other hand, would provide something that blocks up the nose.

Homoeopaths claim that, nowadays, a remedy can be formulated to aid virtually every disorder, including circulatory problems and varicose veins. Although remedies are safe and non-addictive, occasionally the patient's symptoms may briefly worsen. This is known as a 'healing crisis' and is usually short-lived. It is actually a good indication that the remedy is working well.

It is a common misconception that you can just pop along to your local chemist, look up your particular complaint on the homeopathic remedy chart, and begin taking the remedy. If only it were that simple ... Homoeopathic training takes several years, and a lot of knowledge and experience is required before practitioners can decide the correct remedies for complaints other than the very superficial. And, as I mentioned earlier, homoeopathy is specific to each individual person. What works for one person is not likely to work for another. That said, certain of the following remedies are often selected for treating varicose veins:

- carbo vegetabilis – for poor circulation, constipation and varicose ulcers;
- belladonna – for varicose veins that are red, hot, swollen and tender;
- hamamelis – for pain and discomfort from varicose veins, available as a tincture or lotion (the lotion should be applied at night);
- pulsatilla – to treat varicose veins after childbirth;
- lachesis – for painful inflammation in varicose veins of blue colour on the left side of the body;
- arnica – for tenderness, bruising and pain, and often used after varicose vein surgery;
- ferrum metallicum – for varicose veins in pale legs that redden easily;
- calcarea fluorica – to improve the elasticity of vein walls.

Hydrotherapy

In order to stimulate circulation in the legs, it can be of great benefit to alternate between hot and cold baths. To achieve this, you need two buckets that are tall enough to submerge the legs up to the knees. Fill one bucket with water that is comfortably hot and the other with cold or cool water. To each one you can either add two tablespoonfuls of Epsom salts per litre (quart) of water or a few drops of an aromatherapy oil (see pages 95–9). Step into the bucket of hot water for 2–3 minutes, then step into the bucket of cold water for about 30 seconds. Repeat the procedure three times, finishing with a soak in the cold bucket.

To see good results, perform hydrotherapy once a day for 4–6 weeks. People who have diabetes should use warm water, not hot.

Pain and discomfort from superficial varicose veins can be eased by spraying or sponging cold water onto the affected areas.

Hypnotherapy

For several decades it has been known that hypnotherapy is capable of reducing stress, anxiety and phobias. When anxiety about the cosmetic appearance of your varicose veins interferes with your normal routine – with the clothes you choose to wear, for instance – hypnotherapy is an avenue well worth exploring. It can make all the difference to the way you see your physical self.

The reason that more people with cosmetic concerns don't pursue hypnotherapy is its negative media perception. One common fear is that the therapist may, while you are in a trance state, implant dangerous suggestions, or extract improper personal information. I can only stress that patients can come out of the trance at any time – particularly if they are asked to do or say something they would not even contemplate when awake. Malpractice would only have to be brought to light once to ruin the therapist's career.

Hypno*therapy* is actually about the hypnotist using the power of hypnotism for *therapeutic* purposes. The person under hypnosis is in a state of heightened awareness and focused concentration – scientifically measurable by instruments and known as the 'alpha state'. Scientific research has shown this state of mind to be superior for learning, memory recall and training the mind to overcome negative programming, which might include a stressful reaction to unsightly veins. During hypnotherapy, the therapist attempts to remove the emotional response from certain associations. Once that has been done, he or she can help the unconscious mind to focus on stimuli other than the head noises.

After the first session, the therapist may recommend that you purchase an audiotape to allow you to self-hypnotize on a daily basis. Self-hypnosis has been studied on several occasions, and the average improvement rate lies between 60 and 75 per cent.

The Yellow Pages phone book will provide the numbers of several hypnotherapists in your area. The charge is generally reasonable and hypnotherapists tend to be kindly, attentive people.

Massage

The pain and discomfort of varicose veins can be significantly reduced by regular massage. Your trained massage therapist will start at your feet and massage upwards to your thighs and along the lymphatic system to loosen congested blood and other tissues, always stroking upwards towards the heart.

If you allow someone who is not trained in massage therapy to work on your legs, or if you do it yourself, remember that your varicose veins should never receive direct massage. However, a general ankle and leg massage can help to decrease swelling in the veins. In massaging yourself, sit comfortably on a sofa or bed with your legs slightly raised on a pillow. Without touching the veins, apply smooth strokes from the feet to the upper thigh. A daily massage session of about 5 minutes should provide an improvement in 4–6 weeks.

Reflexology

Reflexology, an ancient oriental therapy, was only recently adopted in the Western world. It operates on the proposition that the body is divided into different energy zones, all of which can be exploited in the prevention and treatment of any disorder.

Reflexologists have identified 10 energy channels that begin in the toes and extend to the fingers and the top of the head. Each channel relates to a particular bodily zone, and to the organs in that zone. For example, the big toe relates to the head (that is, the brain, ears, sinus area, neck, pituitary glands and eyes). By applying pressure to the appropriate terminal in the form of a small, special-ized massage, a reflexologist can determine which energy pathways are blocked.

Experts in this type of manipulative therapy claim that all the organs of the body are reflected in the feet. They also believe that reflexology aids the removal of waste products and blockages within the energy channels, improving circulation and lymph gland func-tion. It can therefore be of great benefit in treating varicose veins. Reflexology is certainly relaxing – for the mind and body. Indeed, as well as reducing stress, it can lessen depression.

Many therapists prefer to take full case history before com-mencing treatment. Each session will take up to 45 minutes (the preliminary session may take longer), and you will be treated sitting in a chair or lying down. In treating varicose veins, the points that are usually worked on correspond with the adrenal glands, the parathyroid glands, the digestive system (especially the liver), the spine, the heart and the sciatic nerve.

Relaxation

Long-term frustration and anxiety invariably lead to chronic stress – the state of being constantly 'on alert'. The physiological changes associated with this state (a fast heart-rate, shallow breathing and muscular tension) often persist over a long period, making relaxation very difficult.

Chronic stress can lead to nerviness, hypertension, irritability and depression.

Deep breathing

In normal breathing, we take oxygen from the atmosphere down into our lungs. The diaphragm contracts and air is pulled into the chest cavity. When we breathe out, we expel carbon dioxide and other waste gases back into the atmosphere. But when we are stressed or upset, we tend to use the rib muscles to expand the chest. We breathe more quickly, sucking in shallowly. This is excel-lent in a crisis because it allows us to obtain the optimum amount of oxygen in the shortest possible time, providing our bodies with the extra power needed to handle the emergency. However, some people tend to get stuck in chest-breathing mode. Long-term shallow breathing is not only detrimental to physical and emotional health, it can also lead to hyperventilation, panic attacks, chest pains, dizziness and gastrointestinal problems.

To test your breathing, ask yourself:

1 How fast are you breathing as you are reading this?
2 Are you pausing between breaths?
3 Are you breathing with your chest or with your diaphragm?

A breathing exercise

The following deep breathing exercise should, ideally, be performed daily:

1 Ensure that you are not wearing tight clothing. If you are, changing into something loose-fitting.
2 Make yourself comfortable in a warm room where you know you will be alone for at least half an hour.
3 Close your eyes and try to relax.
4 Gradually slow down your breathing, inhaling and exhaling as evenly as possible.
5 Place one hand on your chest and the other on your abdomen, just below your rib-cage.
6 As you inhale, allow your abdomen to swell upward. (Your chest should barely move).
7 As you exhale, let your abdomen flatten.

... Give yourself a few minutes to get into a smooth, easy rhythm. As worries and distractions arise, don't hang on to them. Wait calmly for them to float out of your mind – then focus once more on your breathing.

When you feel ready to end the exercise, open your eyes. Allow yourself time to become alert before getting up. With practice, you will begin breathing with your diaphragm quite naturally – and in times of stress, you should be able to correct your breathing without too much effort.

Stress-busting suggestions

If you feel stressed about the appearance of your varicose veins or their symptoms, try to put into practice the stress-busting suggestions below. Carrying out at least two or three different ones every day should enable you to cope better with your day-to-day life:

- Smile as often as you can.
- Drive in the slow lane.
- Perform your daily activities at a slower pace (walking, eating, reading, housework, washing the car, doing the crossword puzzle and so on).
- Stop yourself from grimacing.
- Buy a small gift for someone you care about.
- Tell someone you care about how much they mean to you.
- Pay someone a compliment.
- Refer to yourself less frequently in conversation.
- Practise controlling your anger.
- Allow yourself to cry if you feel like doing so.
- Practise assertiveness.
- Listen to music.
- Take a long bath.
- Alter your routine slightly.
- Take a leisurely walk around a park or through woodland.
- Notice nature more (the flowers, birds, trees, rainbows and sunsets).

A relaxation exercise

Relaxation is one of the forgotten skills in today's hectic world. However, learning at least one relaxation technique can counter the stress arising from varicose vein symptoms and anxiety over their cosmetic appearance.

The following exercise is perhaps the easiest:

1 Ensure that you are not wearing tight clothing.
2 Make yourself comfortable in a place where you will not be disturbed. (Listening to restful music may help you relax.)
3 Begin to slow down your breathing, inhaling through your nose to a count of two.

4 Letting your abdomen swell upwards and barely moving your chest, exhale to a count of three, four, five or six.

After a couple of minutes, concentrate on each part of your body in turn, starting with your right arm. Consciously relax each set of muscles, allowing the tension to flow right out ... Let your arm feel heavier and heavier as every last remnant of tension seeps away ... Follow this procedure with the muscles of your left arm, then the muscles of your face, your neck, your stomach, your hips and, finally, your legs.

Visualization

At this point, visualization can be introduced into the exercise. As you continue to breathe slowly and evenly, imagine yourself surrounded, perhaps, by lush, peaceful countryside, beside a gently trickling stream – or maybe on a deserted tropical beach, beneath swaying palm fronds, listening to the sounds of the ocean, thousands of miles from your worries and cares. Let the warm sun, the gentle breeze, the peacefulness of it all wash over you ...

The tranquillity you feel at this stage can be enhanced by repeating the exercise frequently – once or twice a day is best. With time, you should be able to switch into a calm state of mind whenever you feel stressed.

Meditation

Arguably the oldest natural therapy, meditation is the simplest and most effective form of self-help. Dr Herbert Benson of Harvard Medical School has been able to show that meditation tends to normalize blood pressure, the pulse rate and level of stress hormones in the blood. He has proved, too, that it produces changes in brain wave patterns (showing less excitability), and that it strengthens the immune system and endocrine system.

The unusual thing about meditation is that it involves 'letting go', allowing the mind to roam freely. Most of us are used to trying to control our thoughts – in our work, for example – so letting go is not as easy as it sounds.

It may help to know that people who regularly meditate say they have more energy, require less sleep, are less anxious, and feel far 'more alive' than before they did so. Ideally, the technique should be taught by a teacher – but, as meditation is essentially performed alone, it can be learned alone with equal success.

Meditation may, to some people, sound a bit off-beat. But isn't it worth a try, especially when you can do it for free! Kick off those shoes and make yourself comfortable, somewhere you can be alone for a while. Now follow these simple instructions:

1 Close your eyes, relax and practise the deep breathing exercise as described above.
2 Concentrate on your breathing. Try to free your mind of conscious control.
3 Let your mind roam unchecked, and try to allow the deeper, more serene part of you to take over.
4 If you wish to go further into meditation, concentrate on mentally repeating a 'mantra' – a certain word or phrase. It should be something positive, such as 'relax', 'I feel calm' or even 'I am special'.
5 When you are ready to finish, open your eyes and allow yourself time to adjust to the outside world before getting to your feet.

The aim of mentally repeating a mantra is to plant positive thoughts into your subconscious mind. It is a form of self-hypnosis – only you alone control the messages placed there.

Schuessler tissue salts

Schuessler tissue salts (also called mineral tissue salts) are an offshoot of homoeopathy and are thus completely safe. As with most complementary therapies, they can be used in conjunction with conventional medication without any side-effects. Schuessler tissue salts are reputed to be particularly beneficial in a body that is overly acidic, as is the case for people with circulatory disorders. They are also useful for treating minor illnesses from skin conditions to sinus disorders.

The original 12 remedies were isolated by Dr Wilhelm Schuessler, in 1880. The natural ingredients are homoeopathically prepared to a potency that is reputed to allow the cells to rebalance their 'salts' content, in order to restore health. The tiny white tablets dissolve in the mouth, leaving a pleasant taste. There are more than 30 different tissue salts in all, but the most useful for people with varicose veins are:

- magnesium phosphorica: 6X, for acute, cramp-like, spasmodic pains;
- calcarea fluorica: 6X, for bulging and dilated veins, a tendency to varicose ulceration, muscular weakness or bluish discoloration of the tissues;
- ferrum phosphorica: 6X, for vein inflammation red streaks following the course of the vein or throbbing along a vein; it can be used as an alternative to calcarea fluorica.

Schuessler tissue salts are available from health food shops and some chemists.

Yoga

The stretching and relaxation techniques used in yoga can be of particular benefit for people with varicose veins. Positions such as the plough, corpse and half shoulder can improve the circulation and aid drainage of blood from the legs. Moreover, the deep breathing exercises taught in yoga may relieve discomfort by improving oxygenation of the blood.

Useful addresses

Better Life Healthcare
Unit 3, Cuerdean Green Mill
Sherdeley Road
Lostock Hall
Preston
Lancashire PR5 5LP
Tel.: 0800 328 9338
Website: www.betterlifehealthcare.com

A distributor of healthcare products – including support and compression stockings and tights – to members of the general public, private and trade organizations and the NHS.

British Varicose Vein Centre
The Hospital of St John and St Elizabeth
Grove End Road
London NW8 9NH
Tel. 020 7078 3822
Website: www.varicoseveins.co.uk
Email: bvvc@varicoseveins.co.uk

The centre offers private treatment for varicose veins and spider veins. It specializes in varicose-vein treatment under local anaesthetic in an outpatients' department.

Cosyfeet
Foot Shop Ltd
The Tanyard
Leigh Road
Street
Somerset BA16 0HR
Tel.: 01458 447275
Website: www.cosyfeet.com
Email: comfort@cosyfeet.com

For medically approved footwear and other hip-to-toe products, including anti-DVT items, support and compression stockings, waterproof stockings for use in the shower, and so on. Ring or email to order a full catalogue.

National Institute for Clinical Excellence (NICE)
MidCity Place
71 High Holborn
London WC1V 6NA
Tel.: 020 7067 5800
Website: www.nice.org.uk

This independent organization is responsible for providing national guidelines on the promotion of good health and the prevention and treatment of numerous health conditions, including varicose veins. NICE works closely with the NHS and offers guidance on the use of new and existing medicines, treatments and procedures within the NHS.

The Vascular Society
Royal College of Surgeons of England
35–43 Lincoln's Inn Fields
London WC2A 3PE
Tel.: 020 7973 0306
Website: www.vascularsociety.org.uk

This is an internet-based site containing information for people suffering from vascular problems. It gives details of events, fundraising initiatives and successful projects.

The Whiteley Clinic
1 Stirling House
Stirling Road
Guildford
Surrey GU2 7RF
Tel.: 0870 766 1234
Website: www.thewhiteleyclinic.co.uk

This is a private medical facility which specializes in the surgical and non-surgical removal of varicose veins, lymphoedema and peripheral arterial disease.

USA

American Society for Dermatologic Surgery (ASDS)
5550 Meadowbrook Drive
Suite 120
Rolling Meadows
IL 60008, USA
Tel.: 847-956-0900
Website: www.asds.net

Provides information on skin conditions and treatments, together with a list of ASDS members in your area.

Support Hose Store
2300 S. Bell, Suite 2
Amarillo
TX 79106, USA
Tel.: 1-800-515-4271
Website: www.supporthosestore.com

This company offers support and compression stockings manufactured in many different styles by the certified fitters Jobst, Mediven and Sigvaris. It also publishes a regular newsletter, *Leg Health News.*

References

1. Varicose veins – an overview

1. C. J. Evans, P. J. Allan, A. J. Lee, A. W. Bradbury, C. V. Ruckley and F. G. R. Fowkes (1998) 'Prevalence of venous reflux in the general population on duplex scanning: the Edinburgh vein study', *Journal of Vascular Surgery*, 28: 767–76.
2. A. Bradbury, C. Evans, P. Allan, A. J. Lee, C. V. Ruckley and F. G. R. Fowkes (1999) 'What are the symptoms of varicose veins? Edinburgh vein study cross sectional population survey', *British Medical Journal*, 318: 353–6.
3. T. Andrew, T. D. Spector, S. Jeffery (2005) 'Linkage to the FOXC2 region of chromosome 16 for varicose veins in otherwise healthy, unselected sibling pairs', *Journal of Medical Genetics*, 42: 235–9.

6. A nutritional approach to varicose veins

1. Dr Russell Blakelock (1996) *Excitotoxins: The Taste that Kills*, Health Press Books.
2. Dr H. J. Roberts (1995) *Defense against Alzheimer's Disease*, Sunshine Sentinel Press Inc.

9. Vein ligation and stripping

1. J. R. Barwell, C. E. Davies, J. Deacon, K. Harvey and J. Minor (2004) 'Comparison of surgery and compression with compression alone in chronic venous ulceration', *The Lancet*, 363: 1854–9.
2. E. Einarsson, B. Eklof and P. Neglen (1993) 'Sclerotherapy or surgery as treatment for varicose veins: A prospective randomized study', *Journal of Phlebology*, 8: 22–6.
3. Einarsson *et al.* (1993).
4. R. K. Mackenzie, A. J. Lee, A. Paisley, P. Burns, *et al.* (2002) 'Patient, operative and surgeon factors that influence the effect of superficial venous surgery on disease-specific quality of life', *Journal of Vascular Surgery*, 35: 896–902.
5. W. B. Campbell, A. Vijay Kumar, T. W. Collins, K. L. Allington and J. A. Michaels (2003) 'The outcome of varicose vein surgery at ten years: clinical findings, symptoms and patient satisfaction', *Annals of the Royal College of Surgeons of England*, 85: 52–7.
6. Mackenzie *et al.* (2002).

7. K. P. de Roos, F. H. Nieman and H. A. M. Neumann (2003) 'Ambulatory phlebectomy versus compression sclerotherapy', *Dermatologic Surgery*, 29: 221–6.
8. G. Critchley *et al.* (1997) 'Complications of varicose vein surgery', *Annals of the Royal College of Surgeons of England*, 93: 105–10.
9. Einarsson *et al.* (1993).
10. G. Belcaro, M. R. Cesarone, A. Di Renzo *et al.* (2003) 'Foam sclerotherapy, surgery, sclerotherapy and combined treatment for varicose veins: A 10-year prospective randomized controlled trial', *Angiology*, 54; 307–15.
11. Belcaro *et al.* (2003).
12. S. Sarin, J. H. Scurr and P. D. Coleridge-Smith (1994) 'Stripping of the long saphenous vein in the treatment of primary varicose veins', *British Journal of Surgery*, 81: 1455–8.

Further reading

Campbell, B., *Understanding Varicose Veins*. Family Doctor Publications, Poole, 2000.

Goldman, M. P., *Ambulatory Phlebectomy: Basic and Clinical Dermatology*. Marcel Dekker (part of Taylor & Francis), London, 2005.

Goldman, M. P., Bergan, J. J., Guex, J.-J., *Scleropathy: Treatment of Varicose and Telangiectatic Leg Veins*. Mosby Publications, St Louis, Mo., 2006.

Hay, L. L., *Love Yourself, Heal Your Life Workbook*. Hay House Inc., Carlsbad, Calif., 2004.

Musson, R. A., *Varicose Veins and Spider Veins: Myths and Realities*. Zepp Publications, Fairlawn, Ohio, 2001.

Sadick, N. S., *Manual of Scleropathy, 1999*. Lippincott, Williams and Wilkins, Philadelphia, Penn., 1999.

Index